Practical Problems in General Practice

Practical Problems in General Practice

by

Malcolm Fox, MB, CHB, DOBSTRCOG, FRCGP
General Practitioner,
Macclesfield, Cheshire

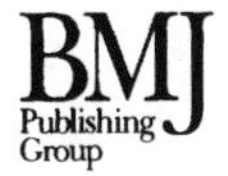

First published in 1997
by the BMJ Publishing Group, BMA House, Tavistock Square, London WC1H 9JR

British Library Cataloguing in Publication Data

A catalogue record for this book is available from the British Library

ISBN 0-7279-1037-X

Typeset, printed and bound in Great Britain by

Contents

Preface

The business of general practice is becoming increasingly complex, with change driven as much by alteration in clinical practice as organisational factors. With the addition of fundholding it is increasingly common for practices to have a multi-million pound turnover and extensive payrolls of clinical and other staff.

This results in general practices which are steadily evolving from simple doctor partnerships to complicated organisations responsible for the delivery and organisation of a wide range of health care. As a consequence, all practitioners are finding that they need to devote a greater proportion of their energy to the non-clinical tasks. Effective management of practices will maximise the value of their clinical services to patients and, importantly, minimise the distraction of doctors from their clinical tasks. Simultaneously it should maximise practice income and ensure the maximum of useful economical expenditure, thus facilitating profitability.

The whole of this process of continuous change is intimidating to existing practitioners, and particularly intimidates new entrants to practice. The composition of the training programmes for practitioners inevitably concentrates primarily on the clinical workload.

This book is mainly aimed at the trainee registrar and the new principal in practice in order to provide them with a basic level of information and education from which further study can develop. It should be useful for the new entrant to practice management and help managers in health authorities understand and guide practices.

There is a degree of provocation in many of the ideas and concepts, which should make the text of interest to established practitioners and managers. It is hoped that this will stimulate further review and education.

MALCOLM FOX
Macclesfield

1: Business planning

The concept of business planning has been seen by practitioners to symbolise the worst aspects of the health services reforms. There is a formal requirement of fundholders to produce a yearly plan and it is an increasing expectancy that all practices will function in the same way, particularly where they are seeking to gain extra resources from the health authority.

This can be seen as a new irritation for established practices but it is not entirely a new process. Applications to banks for finance and negotiation with health authorities in arranging attachments or grants have always needed a description of the intended use and implications for the practice.

The formal definition

A business plan is a statement of the actions and resources required by a business to sustain and develop a discreet area of commercial activity over time.

The business plan as defined can be likened and demystified by comparing the process to a clinical consultation, which commences with an information gathering exercise of determining the signs and symptoms, deciding on the appropriate investigations and then agreeing the most appropriate treatment. It is useful to remember that the science of management tends to surround itself in a mist of almost incomprehensible jargon and abbreviation which has much in common with how the medical world functions.

A simple planning process

- An analysis of current practice activity
- A statement of the organisation's future intentions
- The work and resources needed to achieve the objectives

One of the current fashions in management jargon is referred to as the KISS principle, the interpretation of the acronym being, "Keep it Simple, Stupid". There is an alternative view that this principle is the reverse to what is needed!

The value of planning

Before progressing to the detail of the process, it is worth giving some thought as to the usefulness of business planning. Practices are continuously changing in their personnel, both medical and otherwise, their facilities and resources and the nature of the services they deliver to their patients. Frequently this seems to happen entirely by chance, but in reality it is often planned orally carefully in advance. This is therefore an existing process of business planning. The exercise of formalising the process in writing helps to ensure that all the ramifications and consequences are considered and calculated.

Reasons for writing a plan

- To raise money
- To ensure survival
- To achieve change
- To show commitment
- To establish a common sense of purpose

The relevance of each of the features listed to general practice and concepts of team service are obviously essential to patient care. The process of ensuring survival is being able to continue to operate efficiently and profitably, which has an importance in itself.

When a practice wishes to change any aspect of its activity or organisation it needs to be able to explain the process, how it will be accomplished, and understand the consequences of change. The process of planning helps to keep the necessary drive alive and, along with involving all the people affected, show and develop commitment to a common purpose.

The presentation should present an easily understood picture of current activities, what change it intends to make, and how that will be brought about. It will be a poor plan if it attempts to show that the practice is setting impossible or unrealistic targets.

The effort of developing and writing a business plan which presents a comprehensive picture of current activity and anticipated change, developed by the whole practice is in itself a process which encourages commitment which helps to hold the team together and dynamise its activities. This will help to produce a sense of individual usefulness which can be encouraged and facilitate joint working.

Planning for fundholders

Fundholders business plans have to be produced annually and particularly emphasise the elements contained within the fund. There is a need to report on the usage of public money and the future intentions on expenditure. The detail of this will form part of the business plan, either in the main part or as a specific appendix.

Various people and organisations have a legitimate interest in knowing of a practice's plans for the future in order to represent their own interests, such as the provider organisations and the consumer, represented by Community Health Councils and patient groups. The health authority will be seeking information to ensure the maximum operational and financial efficiency. A skilfully written plan can significantly influence the original agreement to proceed and the level of budget allowed.

Developing and writing the plan

Inevitably the development of a plan will involve some devotion of time by members of the practice. The work can be shared, but it is likely to progress faster and with less strain if a limited number of people are involved in the process of collation and writing. A properly trained and knowledgeable practice manager who is kept fully informed by the partners will be able to create the skeleton on which the detail is built. The manager should also be able to put some flesh and corroborating detail on to the expressed wishes of the whole team.

Crucial elements

- Nominate the writer or writers
- Identify sources of help
- Obtain relevant information
- Incorporate team views
- Continuously consult

Alternatively, the work can be shared by each partner having a dedicated section to complete. This is a useful method of spreading the workload but it has the disadvantage of potentially producing a disjointed plan. As the practice gains confidence in the abilities of its managerial and administrative team when the process has been repeated a few times, there will be a decreasing need of clinicians' time.

Sources of planning assistance

- The intended recipient – defining the format and detail requirements
- Professional medical and managerial colleagues
- Educational courses
- Professional accountants
- Business consultants
- Books and journals.

Each of the sources of planning assistance listed has its advantages and disadvantages and varying degrees of financial implications. Externals are often too easily seen as a quick and pain-free, even if costly, solution. Unfortunately, because they start with little local knowledge, the briefing process is very important, and can almost amount to doing the work internally.

Sources of information

The relevant information needed for the planning process can be extensive but is readily available. It is frequently already being accumulated both within a practice and outside.

Relevant data available within the practice

- Team members and their skills
- List size and demography
- Target achievement and health promotion data
- Accounts
- Patient contact data
- Disease indexes and knowledge of clinical presentations
- Referral information including use of investigation services
- Knowledge of other local health care services
- Results of audit activity
- Prescribing reports (PACT)

This information is then complemented by that made available by the local public health team. This should include local mortality data and what is known about disease prevalence. It will add to the practitioners' knowledge of local occupational health risks. Health visitors are trained to expect to produce a practice profile; these are very useful in providing a range of information on the local community, varying from schools to voluntary organisations, as well as unmet health needs.

Relevant public policy documents

- "Health of the Nation" policy and planning
- Local community care plans
- Health authority policy plans
- Health provider organisation plans

Practitioners will also know how the practice of medicine is changing. This will be detailed and extensive in the primary care field and less so in the secondary and tertiary sectors. National policies are promulgated by professional organisations and bodies and pressure groups continuously canvas practitioners to promote the interests of their members. There is an increasing volume of research and guidance on the effectiveness of health care interventions which has to be taken into account.

Increasingly practices are coming together in groups, usually for audit and commissioning tasks. The outcomes of these processes have a relevance to practice planning and need incorporation.

Emphasis has to be given to the concept of getting the opinions of all of the team members. It is impossible for any individual to have a monopoly of knowledge, even within their own personal field, and all are continuously learning both by experience and more formal education. Nurses from a variety of disciplines can bring useful different perspectives to problems, as equally the receptionists bring knowledge gained in their daily activity within the organisation.

Finding time for planning

As the planning progresses, ideas and concepts will change, become clarified and extended. Confusion and dispute will need to be settled. Very useful to the process of gaining practice views, achieving consensus and motivating partners and staff are Time Outs and Away Days. This is where a group meets separately, usually at a different location from normal practice, to undertake collation and analysis leading to the planning decisions.

These activities are difficult to arrange against the pressures of a heavy clinical demand but can vary from a few hours only, to a prolonged period. Their value can be improved by using a professional facilitator, who should do some advance groundwork preparation and have an idea of the type of outcome needed. On occasions it may be appropriate for such meetings to be predominantly doctor-based, while on other occasions all the disciplines contained within the practice may be involved.

The analytical process

A major process problem of planning is finding how to cope with the vast amount of knowledge, information and opinion. The relevance and importance of each item will vary and not be consistent over a period of time. A frequently recommended process to assist in coping is the SWOT analysis.

The SWOT analysis

- Strengths
- Weaknesses
- Opportunities
- Threats

Strengths

The obvious strengths of a practice are the skills and knowledge of the whole team. The training, qualifications, and organisational and managing skills of the doctors is probably obvious but the extended team all have a contribution to make.

A major strength of practices is the list of registered patients. Generally they are intensely loyal to a particular practice, with a great reluctance to change practices. Practices with a large turnover of patients often have a degree of security, as in inner city areas where new patients can be signed on to the list at a rate fast enough to ensure stability. Local knowledge is a major strength of practices, extending from an intimate knowledge of the patients and their need and use of health care to more demographic information on likely local housing and industrial developments.

Weaknesses

These are likely to be in the gaps in a practice's services and absence of resources. Identified gaps in services may be the non-provision of what is now common practice services, such as asthma clinics. They may also be those clinical problems which present particular problems in the practice, such as an excess of elderly handicapped patients.

The absence of resources may vary from inadequate premises, lack of access to facilities, and inadequate personnel to an inability to fund projects or ideas. Additionally, weaknesses or problems could be specific to the locality, such as the particular social and ethnic mix of the community served creating particular difficulties with expectations and communications.

Opportunities

The opportunities are what is identified by analysing what the practice feels it is able to do to strengthen or maintain its position in serving its patients. These may mean improving some particular aspect of current services. Alternatively, the opportunity may be to influence or finance some other provider to develop a new service.

The knowledge of the particular climate of the health service at the moment can also be an opportunity. This is exemplified currently by the concept of the primary care led health service where plans for joint action by fundholders or coordinated practices acting together in commissioning are very influential.

Threats

This aspect of the analysis should be an honest and rational appreciation of what will stop or limit the practice's ability to carry forward its plans. This covers areas such as the available time of the practice team, its morale, and how motivated it is in particular areas. This may be exemplified by, say, identifying a local problem of health care for travellers but no individual having a particular interest in the issue and therefore needing a lot of effort in motivation. Similarly, if resources such as premises are a principal issue, the absence of suitable alternative obtainable sites will be a threat to delivery and may result in a delayed or altered outcome. Cost and finances will almost inevitably figure at some point in the threats.

Additional threats must include aspects of competition. A practice choosing to try to increase its list size needs to be aware how neighbouring practices are currently functioning. Decisions to develop in-house services can be affected by plans of other local service providers.

The final plan

To have any use and relevance, the final plan should be as clear and concise as possible. The planning cycle is likely to involve yearly editions. These may be reports on progress on past plans or may involve extensive change due to altered priorities.

The presentation

- Scene setting, the mission, and the practice objectives
- Definition of the objectives
- Controlling and monitoring the process
- The strategic context
- Appendices

The final prepared plan needs to be a coherent, readable document, easily understood by those involved in its preparation and delivery and also by an informed outsider. It therefore needs to be concisely written, without explaining every detail and not excessively long. These suggested section headings form a useful skeleton.

Scene setting and the practice mission

This is a general section which encompasses a broad description of current activity and the general philosophical approach of the practice. There should be a brief description of the practice, its immediate past developments and the health, social, and demographic environment in which it functions. It should always offer an explanation of the local difficulties in delivering care.

The term "Mission Statement" often will be regarded as meaningless managerial jargon. However, in this context it does allow the practice to express its fundamental beliefs and attitudes, which can influence outsiders. It may assert a prime role of reactive care or it may offer a desire for more anticipatory care. The majority of practices would want to subscribe to a statement saying that its core value was to help the sick, not to waste its own or others' money and to keep all the practice workers happy.

Practice objectives and the monitoring role

The practice objectives is a list of the intended changes set against continuing arrangements. They will usually, but not inevitably, be descriptions of changes in clinical services. Planned changes in medical staffing, other staff and their recruitment and training, and the practice premises will appear at this point. Similarly this is the place for decisions on relationships with other bodies to be presented, such as a change in referral patterns or a desire to change existing contracts.

All of the objectives need to be accompanied by a statement as to how they will be accomplished. This will include a financial appraisal and an indication as to the likely origin of the resources, the final feature being an estimate of the likely timescale. The important point is that objectives are realistic, although their delivery may well stretch the practice.

This then leads logically to the control and monitoring process. This can be a very specific section where relevant methods of clinical audit are defined. It is more likely to be the place where responsibility for completing the objectives, their sequence, and timing are defined.

The strategic context

The strategic issues affecting the future are the rather less easily measured or defined factors. A potential manpower crisis affecting the recruitment of doctors is less likely to affect a practice with no obvious retirement for five years than one facing the same situation tomorrow. A change of local hospital or secondary care services, such as more day surgery, may affect the practice but the exact degree may not be obvious for a period. The rate at which an area is redeveloped or a new housing development completed may well be unclear.

New medical technology and techniques will always be a major problem somewhat indeterminate in time. The use of keyhole surgery is an example of this, as is the potential explosion of work associated with genetic screening. Further health service structural reorganisation can initially be difficult to assess as to its likely effect.

This is the section to explain a long term phased approach to meeting objectives or an explanation of how policy will be developed in a looser longer term perspective.

Supporting information in appendices

- Relevant financial information
- Analysis of possible changes and their consequences
- Contractual details
- Clinical protocols
- Detail of training and audit consequences
- Job descriptions and staff objectives
- Activity levels
- Resources deployed
- Information technology consequences

Any list of appendices such as suggested in the Box is inevitably both intimidating and incomplete. The good news is that none of these sections should be regarded as mandatory or exclusive. They will, and should, be relevant to many objectives but not all.

There is a temptation to try to make appendices so detailed and voluminous that they appear to be much more important than they are. This can also be a bureaucratic tool to make the writers appear more skilled than is realistic.

The business case

This term is frequently used in the context of business planning and can be confusing. It is best applied to the process of presenting a single issue in great detail, such as may be necessary when applying for discretionary grants or funds. The proposition needs to be expounded fully and accompanied by explicit financial and organisational analysis.

It could be argued that a more appropriate business plan could be made up of a multiple of separate business cases. This is unwise as it will fail to place the specific project within the total context of practice activity.

Project management

This is a useful method of ensuring that a particular task or objective is expeditiously completed. The task is closely defined and then broken down into its constituent parts. Each part then has a time for completion and a named individual responsible for it, the whole having an overall named manager and stated end-point.

Recommended reading

Edwards P, Jones S, Williams S. *Business and health planning for general practice.* Oxford: Radcliffe Medical Press, 1994.

Gray D. *Planning primary care.* Occasional Paper 57. London: RCGP, 1992.

Ham C. *The new National Health Service.* Oxford: Radcliffe Medical Press, 1991.

Huntington J. *Managing the practice, whose business?* Oxford: Radcliffe Medical Press, 1995.

Irving D, Irving S. *The practice of quality.* Oxford: Radcliffe Medical Press, 1996.

2: The optimal practice size

There will always be situations where practice size is determined by a combination of geography and population density effectively mandating a particular practice patient list total. The number of doctors is nearly always capable of some alteration or manipulation. Patient list size and the number and availability of doctors are not inevitably tied together in any practice, but are obviously interrelated in their effect on profitability.

How any patients can a practitioner look after?

Most practitioners believe that the quality of care they deliver is directly related to the amount of time they can spend with each individual patient. Therefore a large list means more difficulty in providing patient services but, despite this general agreement, there is no accepted definition of large. The fundamentally capitation-based payment system of the National Health Service encourages large lists as this produces the largest income.

Advantages of a small list

- The availability of more doctor time for each patient
- Increased ability of the doctor to know each patient
- Reduced doctor stress
- Additional time for health education and promotion work in consultations
- Facilitating medical audit and continuing education

A smaller list should help to provide a longer period for each individual consultation with the opportunity to better understand the patient's problem and properly negotiate the plan of management. The provision of sufficient time has the potential to reduce the risk of mistakes and reduce complaints.

The increasing range of services provided by practitioners is encouraged by changing clinical practice, patient expectation, and the administration. Much health care which was previously provided in hospital is now undertaken by practitioners in a variety of community settings alongside totally new services. Simultaneously the rights of patients are being emphasised and there is continual pressure to provide more convenience services at all hours.

Logically these pressures should result in more practitioners being available with reduced list sizes. This is not occurring and would be an expensive solution. Simultaneously some influential health economists and a few practitioners maintain that list sizes do not need to be reduced and can even be increased. They argue that better organisation and more delegation to non-medical personnel is more appropriate and economic.

Aids to managing a large list

- Developing easily followed clinical policies and protocols
- Maximum delegation of medical tasks
- Skill-mix changes in the primary health care team
- Empowering non-medical staff
- Encouraging direct patient access to non-doctor team members
- Close managerial and clinical audit

All of this is based on the premise that doctor time is a scarce and expensive asset in a practice and should not be wasted on any task that any other staff could undertake. To function in this manner it is necessary to have a fully developed and staffed Primary Health Care Team, which in itself is expensive to operate and house. Additionally this approach is justified by the argument that other team members often have a different range of skills not owned by a doctor. They are also often seen to be more approachable and less intimidating than doctors and, especially in the case of nurses, more closely conform to protocols and policies in their work.

There are additional reasons for a small list size which are sometimes linked to part-time working. Some practitioners prefer a small list in order to allow themselves time to undertake additional work both within and without medicine. Within the practice this can be educational or research work and private practice. Externally it can be a whole range of clinical activities in the hospital and community services and industry as well as operating some other business on a part-time basis.

It is therefore inevitable that there is no agreement on the optimal list size. A frequently quoted number is seventeen hundred (1700), which seems to be a reasonable compromise, but it has to be admitted that there is no research basis for suggesting this number. Taking into account the continuing pressures on practitioners to undertake more work in practice it will probably mean that a practice list of this size can only be managed effectively by using the methodology of those advocating large practice lists as above.

Group practice and partnerships

It is easy to consider these two forms of association as essentially the same when in fact they have some different characteristics which may make them appealing to different practitioners. A group practice can be formed by practitioners working together from jointly managed premises employing some or all the necessary staff together but retaining separate business entities. A group of this type can arrange to provide cover for each other on either a paid or barter basis. This type of arrangement is common in dental practice and is used by a small proportion of general practitioners.

Much more commonly such group working is accompanied by the pooling of income, joint staff, equipment and premises management and the distribution of profits on an agreed basis. This is a true partnership, even though in some circumstances not every item of income is pooled.

How large a group or partnership?

About three-quarters of all United Kingdom practitioners work in partnerships or groups. This inevitably brings another dimension to the doctor's professional life which in itself causes additional work. Simply, single-handed practice facilitates rapid decision making and administration whereas working together involves the use of time and effort in organisation and communication.

Advantages of working together

- Facilitates relief cover – off-duty, education, holiday and sickness
- Facilitates peer review and constrains abnormal professional behaviour
- Gives immediate personal support.
- Allows the development of individual specialist knowledge and skills
- Makes feasible the employment of a range of staff with different skills
- Allows economies of scale in practice staff and premises

The view earlier this century of the individual family doctor always being available personally 24 hours each day is no longer tenable. Quite correctly, doctors see themselves now as needing adequate relaxation away from the pressures of work and being entitled to a life apart from their profession. Most now have minimal domestic support and both wish and need to be intimately involved in the care of their families and homes whatever their sex.

Permanent working in partnership or group arrangements allows the rational planning of duty rosters and holidays without the anxieties about locum availability, quality and costs. Similarly, this method of work provides cover in case of sudden or any other type of illness, avoiding the chance that an ill doctor will persevere in trying to work, putting both the patients and the doctor at further risk.

The impact of joint working on clinical standards

When doctors work together in association in the same place there is always a degree of discussion about patients. This can vary from the hand-over of a particular case, say caused by a holiday, to the gossip type of discussion when meeting together formally or more usually informally. The usual sharing of records and lists gives individuals opportunities to learn from the actions of other team members. Despite the informality and chance nature of these contacts they tend to encourage and vitalise good practice. They ensure that it is not possible to stagnate and that there is a regular infusion of new knowledge.

At a more formal level, working together usually involves making some loose agreements or developing consensus on the management of common problems. The effect of this is a degree of pooling of knowledge and information which results in mutual education. Additional joint work on clinical audit and formal continuing education is also possible and improves clinical performance.

Personal support

The practice of medicine is stressful where all are faced daily with patient tragedy and distress. Involvement in patient care frequently carries with it a heavy load of responsibility and emotional entanglement of a humanitarian type. It is recognised that, as a consequence of this pressure, doctors have high levels of depression, drug misuse, and alcoholism. The opportunity to unload anxieties and discuss difficulties hence obtaining peer support eases this problem. Caring colleagues working together can often detect the early signs of stress and illness and facilitate help.

Development of specialisation

Inevitably individual practitioners will have an increased level of knowledge or interest in some areas of practice which is easier to develop and use within a group. There are a number of areas in clinical practice where there is a need to see a sufficient number of patients or practice a procedure frequently to maintain or increase skills. These can be exemplified by diabetic care or the insertion of intra-uterine contraceptive devices. In other situations one doctor taking a more detailed interest in administrative areas such as staff training or financial affairs can be useful.

Care needs to be taken that specialism does not result in the loss of expertise of other team members. It is a particular problem when applied to clinical problems that are common.

Economies of scale

A small practice will usually only be able to afford to employ a small number of staff. This means that they have to try to find multiply skilled staff or employ a larger number of individuals in small amounts of part-time activity thereby increasing the problems of cohesive working. A group of practitioners is able to employ more staff and can generally more easily obtain the services of specialised individuals and therefore provide a wider range of services.

The surgery premises can also be an expensive resource if not used intensively. Depending on the detail, the costs of almost everything supplied and used by the practice can be reduced by larger scale purchasing. Expensive equipment, whether clinical or other, is more economical when used intensively and the purchase cost shared.

Personal lists and practice lists

As a compromise between the apparent two extremes of single-handed practice and group practice, an organisation of clearly separated personal lists within some type of group working is a satisfactory option for some. This can be done within a partnership quite happily. The personal list does enable close and intimate mutual knowledge of doctors and patients and is good for the continuity of care.

Personal lists do risk losing some of the advantages of group practice of mutual education and peer review unless managed carefully. This problem can be minimised by extra effort at comparative clinical audit processes. The operation of personal lists within a group or partnership should not affect the ability to gain from economies of scale.

The isolated practitioner

Genuinely isolated practice can generally do nothing about the number of patients resident locally and therefore the list size, but sometimes there are options in extending the medical manpower of the practice.

One of the few generally welcomed changes of the 1990 contract was the Associate Practitioner scheme. In its present form this allows for two single-handed practitioners whose main surgeries are at least 10 miles apart to share jointly the services of an additional doctor. Effectively the cost of this doctor is paid by the health authority and provides cover for off-duty, holiday, study leave, and sickness.

Some other of the lesser known provisions of the regulations of the health service can be helpful to some individuals in some isolated situations. If a practitioner is aware of an unemployed doctor, suitably qualified, living in the locality who cannot obtain employment and applies for that person to be admitted to the practice as a partner, even if the area is designated as over-doctored, then the health authority has to put the application to the Medical Practices Committee. This statutory body will frequently exercise discretion in this situation and allow the additional doctor to be admitted to partnership.

Similarly, an application for an additional partner, where that new doctor is a member of the existing principal's family, can be approved in the same manner.

The economics of taking these courses of action are problematic because there remains the obligation to ensure that the share of the lowest earning partner is at least one-third of the highest.

Isolated practices can also use the Retainer Scheme to reduce their onerous workload subject to the availability of such a person locally. The direct cost to the practice is minimal and this is further discussed in the chapter on part-time working.

Are some practices too large?

As in most things in life, there cannot be any easily provided ideal. Compromises have to be made and individuals will have decide on their own priorities and match them against what is available.

Too large a group greatly increases the management problem and communications difficulties of all types. Whilst there are examples of successful very large practices, experience is tending to show that the favoured size is in the area of four to six practitioners. In group working this probably means that any individual practitioner will have a good knowledge of his or her own list and accumulate over the years some useful baseline knowledge of most of the patients who have been registered with the practice for some years. A group of this size can give good mutual support for off-duty and also for clinical activity. At this size it should be possible for all the practitioners to meet personally on a daily basis.

This size of group has sufficient economy of scale to allow the employment of well-trained specialised staff on a full-time or adequate part-time basis. It is also of sufficient size to make the best economic sense in the operation of the practice premises and equipment.

The problem of changing practice size

It is not unusual for practices to find themselves faced with external activity which pressurises change or to wish to initiate change themselves. This is not an easy process and problems arise. Large population number changes in localities can arise both from redevelopment reducing the local population and from new housing development. Established practices need always to be aware of what is being planned locally and the district plans produced by local planning authorities can give advance warning as can the usual notices of planning applications. A local housing development as small as fifty houses at an average population density of 2.4 persons per household may pressurise a practice heavily. Equally the demolition of a local high density housing complex could be disastrous.

The appropriate response will always need to be carefully developed and discussed with the health authority. It is not reasonable simply to expect practices to accept extra patients when they do not wish to do so and encouragement to develop another local practice can be a better option. Very major support may be needed to cope with the variations imposed by redevelopment schemes.

A practice may consider its current list size to be too large and wish to make a reduction. A withdrawal of service from a large group of patients without careful planning and negotiation is likely to be disastrous in public relations terms, antagonise other local doctors and the health authority. A planned approach using advance warning and a staged process would be more understandable and sensible. List size may always be reduced by the process of not registering new patients. This can be a slow process in areas of low turnover with little appreciable benefit in the short term. Taking this approach will need a policy which addresses extensions to existing patient families, covering new-born children, new spouses or partners, and grandparents coming to live in the area.

Attracting additional patients

Deliberately aiming to recruit extra patients to increase the practice list size is surprisingly difficult and a slow process unless much new building of residential accommodation is taking place in the area. Patients are generally extremely loyal to practices and their turnover is mainly determined by changes of address.

Attractive premises and the availability of an individual doctor well known in the community is probably the most successful advertisement. Personal doctor involvement in general local community activity, whether sporting and recreational or charitable and public service, certainly creates a useful image. Discrete contact with local estate agents may be helpful but care has to be taken to avoid exceeding the ethical guidelines. The health authority and the local Community Health Council should be informed as patients newly arriving in an area often contact them for information on local practices. Occasionally adjacent practices are pleased to see the development or extension of others in order to relieve their personal load.

Adding a new partner

The major decision of taking on an additional doctor is currently quite difficult. As most pay is capitation-based and basic allowances so small, the existing partners will inevitably face a reduced income. This can be accepted if it results in less individual work but will be complicated by personal financial stress which will vary between doctors.

This means that any such decision has to be accompanied by some serious financial calculations and a plan rapidly to maximise practice income. Policies resulting in the provision of more "Fee for Item of Service" activities and external work are the most promising. An initial period of part-time work can be useful and extended later but will only appeal to some applicants. Another solution is to employ an additional doctor on an assistant basis but care then has to be taken to make the terms of service attractive and financially feasible to both employer and employee.

Recommended reading

Gilligan C, Lowe R. *Marketing and general practice*. Oxford: Radcliffe Medical Press, 1994.

Greig D. *Teamwork in general practice*. Tunbridge Wells: Castle House Publications, 1988.

Marsh G. *Efficient care in general practice*. Oxford: Oxford University Press, 1991.

Pratt J. *Practitioners and practices, a conflict of values*. Oxford: Radcliffe Medical Press, 1995.

Pringle M, Bilkhu J, Dornan M, Head S. *Managing change in primary care*. Oxford: Radcliffe Medical Press, 1994.

Sanderson A. *Income generation in general practice*. Oxford: Radcliffe Medical Press, 1991.

3: Developing practice premises

Why are good premises important?

General practice has changed markedly from the days when the surgery was a place only used for a part of each day to the current situation where the premises are the point from which most of an increasingly sophisticated range of services is delivered throughout most of every day. The premises are also the potential base for all the members of the Primary Health Care Team. There is no doubt that the practice of whatever size with adequate premises is better able to deliver good patient services.

An additional major reason for good premises is that they will act as an advertisement for the people working in the practice and its services. Dingy, poor looking premises demoralise patients and encourage them to view those who work within them and the services provided as inferior.

Characteristics of the ideal premises

- Adequate size
- In the best geographical position
- Considerate of patient transport needs
- Functional disabled access
- Attractive to patients
- Good working environment
- Capable of change

How big is adequate?

Individual opinions on the ideal size of practice premises are likely to differ depending on the extent to which individual doctors feel their own need for protected personal space. As practitioners increasingly spend the majority of their time delivering services from their consulting room, a reasonable starting point is individual consulting rooms and a decision as to whether they need separate examination rooms.

Depending on the size and functions of the team further clinical rooms will be needed, especially if there is any special equipment to be housed or the need for a different ambience, such as for counselling. Almost inevitably the treatment room will be the home of the practice nurse and the place for minor surgery and dressings. If more than one nurse is employed, further rooms could be needed, especially as practice nurses and nurse practitioners function in a quasi-medical consulting and examining role.

Administrative space, including that needed for the storage of records, must also have a high priority, as does the housekeeping functions of kitchens, rest rooms, library, meeting rooms, and stores. Staff need toilet facilities, statutory for separate sexes if a large number are involved, and changing facilities. Finally there is the size of the waiting area or areas. These need to be spacious enough to allow for patients waiting to see other members of the team, and for their escorts and families.

The regulations mandate maximum sizes for consulting rooms and so on, and also the number and type of rooms. This is mainly for the purposes of grants and rent and rates reimbursement. It is not wise to rely on these recommendations as they have not been adequately amended to allow for the changes in practice in the past twenty years and should be regarded as the minimum if at all possible.

Improvement or new building?

Whilst some practices have existed in the same place and building for many years, recently many completely new premises have been built or acquired. The best geographic position for a practice must be one with which existing patients are familiar, has good public transport links and has parking facilities for their use as well as staff. The adjacent presence of other health care providers such as chemists, opticians, dentists, and chiropodists can be a bonus.

Those with disabilities in our community are insistently making their requirements known. Inevitably they will be heavy users of the service and therefore their needs have to be taken into account by providing wheelchair access, disabled toilets, aids for the visually impaired and assistance for the deaf.

Consideration for the needs of the disabled will also partially address the needs of mothers with prams and buggies, although they will also need a secure pram park. Separate waiting facilities for young families with changing and nursing facilities is an enormous benefit and can avoid friction with some of the more frail patients.

Taking all these factors into account will probably result in a decision in favour of new building rather than the inevitable compromises involved in improvements. The planning of alterations will still need to consider all the above factors.

What is the value of good design?

Spending limited practice finance on producing attractive looking premises both internally and externally can be falsely regarded as wasteful. As our society has developed there has been a growth in vandalism and a cavalier attitude to the value of what is apparently public property. However it has become obvious that this poor behaviour can be ameliorated by providing a comfortable attractive environment and there are wide ranges of fittings and decor specially created with heavy, and possibly destructive, use in mind but which are still pleasant. The clean external attractiveness of the premises helps guide both new and old patients to the surgery and expresses pride in the practice which is good for the morale of staff and patients.

The characteristics of a good working environment are a comfortable level of warmth, cleanliness, brightness, good ventilation, and illumination. It must not be crowded or unnecessarily cluttered and noise should be limited as much as possible.

Building for future needs will undoubtedly increase the costs of any project, but it is now very unlikely, with the present pace of change of health care, that any premises will continue to be adequate for more than ten years. Architects, designers, and builders have developed techniques which ease the processes of future adaptation and extension and these possibilities should be included in their initial briefing.

The rent and rates reimbursement scheme

This scheme should, in theory, make it easy for any practice in any part of the country to finance adequate premises. In reality it is a system which has a number of pitfalls. The first is that reimbursement is limited to what the health authority deems to be adequate space, which is usually the minimum space specified in the regulations, and is likely not to coincide with practitioner's views.

The second drawback is the role of the District Valuer. This is a government officer, not in the health service, who sets the notional rents when the premises are owned by the practice or determines what would be a reasonable rent if the practice is a tenant. Frequently that opinion can be at significant variance with other local agents and not bear much relationship to building costs. It is open to practices to dispute these assessments and this should be done whenever feasible, preferably employing an independent agent known to have expertise in the field.

Who owns the premises?

The major problem of being a tenant in any premises is one of security; for an owner it is raising the necessary finance, this being compounded by the problem of significant local variation in land and building costs whatever the arrangement.

Possible practice landlords

- Health authorities
- Specialised financiers
- Local authorities
- Commercial property developers
- Housing developers
- Professional colleagues

Health centres and similar

Until recently one of the most common forms of practice tenancy was renting – sometimes at less than a commercial rent – space in a health centre owned by and shared with a health authority. No new centres of this sort are being built and there is continuing pressure to sell those in existence to the tenant practices or to outright commercial owners. Unfortunately they have gained a reputation of being badly and inflexibly maintained by their owners and tenant practices have been denied development funding from other sources. They did, however, provide better premises than could otherwise be obtained or funded, especially in high cost areas such as inner cities.

Newer versions of these centres are now being offered to practices on a more commercial basis by health authorities, as under the Inner London "Tomlinson" schemes and other Primary Health Care Resource Centre initiatives, usually in major cities. In some areas redundant parts of hospital facilities are being offered to practices on a similar basis. Taking part in these newer schemes usually involves some degree of ownership and can involve other users being tenants. Within these schemes practices can have access to development grants and are able to deploy fundholding savings.

Specialist financiers

The government body with the role of providing specialist financial services to general practice was sold to the Norwich Union group of companies who continue to build and lease practice premises as well as providing financial services. There are several insurance agencies which concentrate on the medical profession and these can offer financial deals often linked to life assurance and pension plans. Some of the major banks also have initiatives on finance specially aimed at practitioners which can be initially approached through normal banking channels.

Local authorities

In some localities, where major redevelopment sponsored by local authorities is occurring, special arrangements may be available. Grants have been made to practices under inner city initiatives and City Challenge schemes. The purchase or lease of land can be facilitated, sometimes on advantageous terms, when the availability of a practice is thought to be socially desirable. Premises made redundant due to changed circumstances, such as former schools or churches, can also be sold or leased.

Property and private housing developers

Established practices are regarded as relatively safe tenants by commercial developers who may build or alter to meet specific practice requirements. The rent sought will be commensurate with their own financial risk and the values of other commercial leasing in the area. The presence of a practice in a particular location may also help to attract other tenants such as chemists and can be used as a bargaining aid. Rents which are regarded as reasonable by the District Valuer are reimbursable in full under the rent and rates scheme.

Where major new private housing developments are occurring, the builders may well be seeking to enhance the general attractiveness by having a range of services and facilities on site. Occasionally they are prepared to develop practice premises for lease in these circumstances or facilitate other advantageous arrangements.

Colleagues as landlords

A common form of tenancy arrangement for practice premises is where the ownership is in the hands of one or more members of the practice but not every partner. At first sight this may not appear to be a tenancy but the cautions listed below are just as relevant. Too often this is an informal arrangement with vague terms which can hinder maintenance, alteration, and use. A proper contract needs to be used with the help of solicitors and property agents to give sensible protection to both parties.

Tenancy problems

Being a tenant will inhibit the practice's ability to decide and act for itself and most changes and even simple maintenance may need negotiation with the owner. Most owners will be seeking a profitable rent related to their investment and it is normal to set rents for an initial period and then review them every three years. Ownership may change without the knowledge of the tenant practice and the balance of power may well lie with the owner. It can be difficult or impossible to obtain health service development funding with an insecure tenancy.

Any tenancy arrangement, even within a practice, will certainly need the assistance of property agents and lawyers to ensure security, probity, and detailed specification of the tenant's rights and obligations. With in-house ownership this should also include some form of a right to buy in specified circumstances, such as at retirement or on the death of the owning partner or partners.

The problems of owner occupation

As practice premises have improved and the range of services provided changes, becoming more complex and expensive, owning doctors have been involved in larger financial borrowing arrangements. This is intimidating, and there are limits as to the amount of capital borrowing which can be financed from earnings. Taken to extreme limits this can deter new partners from joining a practice and can result in retiring partners not being able to sell their shares. There is also the problem of negative equity so obvious in recent years where the general fall in property values has affected practices. Expensive redevelopment of premises rarely gives an equivalent rise in total value and can only be justified against long term inflation or increased earning capacity.

Shared ownership of premises must be covered within the practice agreement and specify individual shares. The method of valuing and the action to be taken when partners join or leave must also be covered. It is unwise to specify particular mortgage or financial arrangements as these are likely to differ for individuals according to their current career point. The differential allocation of ownership on a unequal basis may be a useful interim stage, but anything that does not eventually result in equality of ownership paralleling profit sharing tends to store discord for the future.

The purchase of a share or the whole of practice premises has been seen as a good long term investment realisable at retirement subject to adequate maintenance. Most financiers regard practitioners and practices as relatively safe for investment but they are wary of excessive capital investment.

These complexities are much more problematic as career moves continue to increase. They were much more suitable when practitioners joined a practice for life and could be managed over a period of many years.

Finding a mortgage

Mortgages and loans are available from a variety of sources, but mainly from banks and other commercial lending institutions such as building societies and finance companies. A mortgage is characterised by the lender having a right to take a legal ownership of the property if there is any default on payment. All lenders will want some form of security and will need sight of the practice accounts to ensure that there was reasonable expectation of repayment or a well-developed business plan explaining the effect of the investment on profitability. Different finance sources will inevitably offer terms that differ on interest rates, whether fixed or variable, period of repayment, necessary security, and whether they are willing to lend to all or individual partners according to their needs. There is no alternative for the prospective borrower other than to shop around for the widest range of detailed competing quotations.

A major decision which is difficult to make is whether to link the borrowing closely to an insurance or pension deal. Insurers often offer seemingly easy access to money but the associated deal can be expensive and does not offer the taxation advantages which used to be available. Pension linked deals must be treated with caution as they can involve relinquishing some of the advantages of index linked superannuation. Again the need is for a variety of quotations and careful attention to detail.

Other sources of finance

Cost rent schemes

Where a practice is acquiring new premises, or making major alterations to existing premises, there can be available support from the health service in a "cost rent scheme". This is where the notional rent is foregone in part or wholly and an alternative payment is made to the practice equivalent to the interest charge on the capital borrowed. This is usually at a variable rate as set from time to time by the authorities based around current interest rates. This system is available subject to the consent of the responsible health authority and has to be negotiated in advance of commencing the works. The total amount available for these schemes is cash-limited and agreement is not inevitable.

Additional financial support

- Improvement grants
- Fundholding savings
- Listed building grants
- Becoming a landlord

Improvement grants

On a discretionary basis health authorities can make grants to practices for a wide range of premises and equipment purposes. These are limited to two-thirds of the project value and subject to prior approval. The money available for this use is increasingly restricted and therefore application needs to be pursued vigorously and may involve delaying or modifying plans

Using fundholding savings

Practices which have embarked on fundholding and managed to create savings have been allowed to use them as a source of funding for premises improvement on the basis of providing more suitable arrangements for patient care. This is now being controlled more carefully than initially but acquisition of new and extended premises has been made in this way. Where a practice is providing secondary care services on the practice site, then any necessary premises alterations can be so financed. Otherwise, it is arguable that the practice is profiting from fundholding by increasing its capital asset.

Listed buildings

There are a surprising number of practices located in listed buildings and in some circumstances local authorities can assist in their maintenance and development by grants. The local authority planning office will be aware of the availability of grants and must be consulted anyway as alterations to such premises can be severely restricted.

Becoming a property developer

For a variety of reasons a number of other businesses wish to be based on practice premises or immediately adjacent. The leasing of spare space or the deliberate creation of extra space or facilities for leasing can generate practice income. Almost always a retail pharmacist can be found who is prepared to rent an on-site shop if the practice is of a reasonable size. Chiropodists, physiotherapists, dentists, and retailers of aids for the handicapped may also be interested. Local community health provider trusts and social services departments may also find it useful to rent space on a practice site.

Managing a change of premises

A seemingly simple move from old to new premises can be complex and require a significant amount of planning and involve extra staff costs. Where premises are being redeveloped whilst in use, the transition is complicated by extra problems. Advance thought has to be given to maintaining patient care and access. Allowance has to be made for temporary interim arrangements, even temporary buildings, and contractor problems such as noise, extra cleaning and invasion of privacy. The practice needs to plan carefully with the designers, architects, and builders and ensure that each stage is logical and safe for contractors, staff, and patients. Extra staff costs will always be incurred and the total cost of the scheme can be inflated by these considerations.

Recommended reading

Chisholm J (ed.). *Making sense of the rent scheme.* Oxford: Radcliffe Medical Press, 1992.

Ellis N. *Making sense of general practice.* Oxford: Radcliffe Medical Press, 1994.

Gordon P, Hadley J (eds). *Extending primary care.* Oxford: Radcliffe Medical Press, 1996.

4: Part-time working arrangements

The first problem in this area is deciding what is the difference between part-time and full-time working. Full-time is easiest defined as an individual practitioner who provides services to patients which meets the 26 hour commitment of the terms of service for general practitioners and also plays a full and equal part in the out of hours commitment and organisation of the practice. The current regulations specify that the 26 hours should be spread over five working days and normally delivered for 42 weeks in the year. It follows from this that any other arrangement is part-time.

Varieties of part-time working

- Twenty-six hour commitment principal regularly working less than five days
- Three-quarter time (19 hour) principal in a partnership
- Half-time (13 hour) principal in a partnership
- Part-time work as an assistant
- Retainer scheme as an assistant
- Part-time registrar (trainee) post

It is impossible to work as a part-time principal in any type of practice, unless the individual works in a partnership. It is possible to have a part-time contract as a sole principal where an assistant or assistants is employed to cover the remainder of the commitment.

The health authority can, on a discretionary basis, allow an individual to deliver a 26 hour commitment over less than five days. This is always in the circumstances where work being undertaken on the fifth day is for the benefit of the health service, such as hospital work, medical teaching or research. Whilst this arrangement may commend itself to some, it is potentially disastrous if the individual is attempting to do five days general practice in four days. The addition of the usual out of hours duties plus an additional day's work each week brings the inevitable risk of overwork by the individual and discord in the practice.

Reasons for part-time working

- Practice driven
  - Skill shortage
  - List size
- Personally driven
  - Family commitments
  - Outside interests
  - Age
  - Health problems

Part-time partners

The usefulness of the three-quarter time and the half-time partnership arrangements is greatly affected by the reasons for an individual wanting such an arrangement. When this is being organised so that the individual can reduce work commitments, say prior to retirement or on health grounds, and is meeting their needs then all is well. Equally where this releases an individual to undertake other medical activity, such as teaching, research or hospital work, there are few problems.

Major problems start to arise when an individual feels forced to accept such arrangements on a basis of no other option. Part-time status can be associated with marginalisation and a lack of status in relationships within the team and also with regard to patients. Often female practitioners find this sort of arrangement is the only possibility compatible with other domestic and child care responsibilities. Similarly there may be an element of duress when this is the only local job on offer. Other partners therefore need to approach this with care and clearly detail the working arrangements and definitely not expect to offer part-time pay and expect a full-time commitment.

Essential detail in a part-time agreement

- Working hours and days of attendance
- On-call responsibilities
- Holiday rights and arrangements
- Maternity leave rights
- Sick leave rights
- Study leave arrangements
- Detail of administrative responsibilities
- Freedom to undertake work outside the partnership and retain earnings
- Expectations of providing cover in the absence of another partner
- Provision to revise the agreement at fixed intervals

Part-time partners and practice shares

The four-day full-time arrangement and the two different part-time partnership arrangements apply to the general practice contract with the health authority, which means that the internal partnership arrangement can be different. Sometimes the apparent absentee can make sufficient additional earnings which, if added to the partnership pool, can justify the retention of a full partnership share. This should be subject to very careful agreement of the partners with some fixed agreement to review the arrangement at intervals to allow for changes in income and circumstances to be considered.

Part-time assistantship

This has the attractions and disadvantages of an employed status, whether full- or part-time. Being salaried results in the ability to attend, perform a service, and claim payment for fixed hours of work with a contract of employment. Often this status can avoid much of the administrative and financial problems of partnerships. There is no obligation to invest capital in buying premises and equipment, and it may also be suitable for reasons of personal convenience on hours and place for a period in a career. The main problem of long-term work of this kind is the institutionalisation of an inferior status.

Any assistant should have a contract of employment similar to that for any other practice employee. It needs additionally to specify the same areas as those listed above for part-time partners. Employment as an assistant entitles the employee to full protection under the relevant employment legislation up to and including industrial tribunals if the hours of employment meet the minimum specified.

Can a partner be salaried?

The term salaried partner is used for a limited partnership arrangement where the individual is guaranteed a fixed level of income. This can be satisfactory if it is for a defined period of, say, a year between an assistant status and full profit sharing partnership. A longer period effectively becomes a salaried position without any of the normal employment legislation protection.

It is open to the Inland Revenue and the social security department to challenge this arrangement. Such a challenge could result in financial penalties to the practice if the appropriate officers decided that this was a tax avoidance device. Additionally, it has to be borne in mind that in any partnership the regulations insist that the most junior partner should earn at least one-third as much as the largest partner's income when full time. For three-quarter time partners, they should have a practice income share of at least a quarter of that of the highest earner. For half-time, the appropriate minimum is a one-fifth of the largest partner's earnings.

The retainer scheme

This scheme is intended to help doctors who can only work for a limited time commitment, say for family reasons, to maintain their contact with professional work and their personal skills. The regulations specify that this should not exceed two sessions per week and should have an educational content. Any work undertaken by the individual in practice in excess of two sessions breaches the terms. This is a much abused system but it is very useful for some doctors. The review of individuals on these schemes is the responsibility of the Regional Advisers in General Practice and there are now signs that appropriate policing is being developed. The developing shortage of practitioners probably means that in future there may not be as many willing to take on these arrangements.

Part-time registrars

There is a well-developed and regulated system of part-time training for general practice which allows the in practice period to be spread over two years. This has to be acceptable to the individual's trainer and the Regional Adviser. The European Union has recently developed new regulations on part-time training which insist that in both years the trainee should undertake 60% of the full-time commitment and also have a period of full-time education.

How useful is a part-timer?

There are views in medicine that anyone working less than full time cannot retain full competency. This is not borne out by experience, where part-time doctors usually deliver far more than their personally contracted minimum and many practices could not function without them.

In general terms, the practice list size determines the size of the doctor workforce and simple arithmetic can determine the need for a part-timer. A practice can also benefit from additional doctor time provided by a part-timer with special skills, such as minor surgery or contraceptive services. Such an individual may allow a practice to deliver services which otherwise might be neglected or denied to the local population.

Problems for the individual

It is a sad reflection on the profession that frequently part-time practitioners find themselves the victims of a variety of abuses. This has an extra dimension of abuse when one considers the fact that the majority of part-timers are female and advantage is taken of their sometimes limited mobility and time availability.

Major areas of abuse

- Unfair employment terms
- Inadequate income
- Limited continuity of patient care
- Inability to influence practice actions and policies

The combination of a full professional career with domestic responsibilities and child rearing will be too great a load for most, but need only be a part of the whole of their professional lives. Both male and female doctors can find part-time work most suitable to their circumstances if they have any sort of dependent relative for whom they personally care. Doctors who are incapable of full-time work because of illness problems and or ageing can often continue to contribute effectively to the totality of practice patient care. All of these individuals can bring experience to a practice and enhance its knowledge base and understanding of patient problems. If the exact terms of the relationship are developed and stated explicitly as detailed above, then most abuse and exploitation will be avoided.

Combining two or more jobs

Sometimes a doctor will wish to practise on a part-time basis in order to pursue some alternative outside interest of a non-medical type or even a separate medical post. As a minimum within a practice there needs to be a degree of openness to ensure that there is no clash of interest or any activity likely to bring the practice into disrepute. Most partnership agreements specify the extent to which individual partners are responsible for their own financial affairs and limits their personal ability to mortgage or use as security the earnings and assets of the practice. Additional legal advice may well be needed.

Restrictive covenants

On occasions part-time partners and employed doctors can find themselves being put under pressure to put up with unfair terms by the use of so-called "Restrictive Covenants". These are arrangements which are written in a manner that appears to block any local move to other practices or independent practice. These can seem very intimidating, but it is up to the employer to try to enforce the restrictions through the courts. The courts increasingly regard such covenants as unfair restrictions on trade and employment and tend to find in favour of the individual. Difficulties in these areas can be ameliorated by seeking the help of the BMA Industrial Relations Officers and the mediation of LMC Secretaries operating in their pastoral role.

"We have a lady doctor to do that"

Part-time work can be unsatisfactory if it does not cover the whole of the range of general practice patient contacts. The unspecified duties which result in a part-timer – often female – just providing some cervical cytology and contraceptive services can be quite demotivating, as can the inability to follow through and see the outcome of a complex problem. If a practice wants or needs specific expertise, then this should be specified from the outset and terms negotiated appropriately.

Valuing a part-time colleague

All practices develop systems and policies whether it be about clinical activity, such as referral or prescribing, or organisation, such as the role of the practice staff. Both the apparent status of less authority and time availability can result in a greatly diminished ability to contribute in these areas. The sensible employing practitioner must facilitate and heed the contribution of the part-timer in order to obtain the best value from the employee, which will in turn help the practice and its patients.

Job-sharing

This is a useful arrangement whereby two practitioners jointly take on the work and contract responsibilities of a full-time practitioner and divide the work between themselves on a mutually convenient basis. In the context of a partnership the job sharers should have a joint income at least one-third of the largest.

The two sharers need to have clearly defined relationships between themselves and with the rest of the partnership. Individual hours of availability and handover arrangements are crucial. Two job sharers cannot be expected to provide their own holiday, sick leave, and maternity leave cover unless this is clearly specified and mutually agreed at the outset. It cannot be expected that two job sharers will provide more input to the practice or its patients than a single individual.

Problems can arise over the appointment and resignation of one of the sharers. This form of working arrangement depends, more than most, on good personal relationships, with understanding of each other's needs within the pair. In the context of a partnership clear arrangements need to be made at the outset as to the consequences of one of the pair leaving and his or her replacement. It can be argued and arranged that this is solely the responsibility of the remaining sharer but, usually, other partners will want a say on any incoming individual's suitability. The partnership agreement needs to state clearly the process and action if no suitable replacement is available.

These arrangements for job sharing are very useful for some individuals but not necessarily for the whole of their professional careers. Again, advance thought has to be given as to how this arrangement within a partnership can change as and when necessary.

Part-time work as a locum

Working as a locum can be a useful act both for the individual and for practices. For the individual it has a degree of in-built insecurity, with no specified off-duty or holiday, sickness or maternity pay. The rate charged and paid has to reflect these additional costs and risks and the provision which needs to be made for transport, telephones, and medical defence. The development of an acceptable clientele of employers by the locum can be a difficult process, with individual practices having widely different expectations and arrangements. There is consolation in the fact that there always appears to be a surfeit of available locum work.

Some individuals find this a useful temporary stage in their careers whilst others prefer the personal flexibility of being able to choose time, place, and hours on a more permanent basis, sometimes combined with other medical or non-medical activity. Additionally, personal circumstances affect the individual's ability to take on some of the longer-term opportunities and a wide geographical spread.

The long-term relationship of an individual as a locum to a particular practice can become defined as employment, which results in the acquisition of employed rights and also the normal taxation and social security obligations.

Part-time working and medical indemnity insurance

Whatever type of part-time working is undertaken, individual doctors, and their employers, need to ensure that they have full medical defence cover and that their General Medical Council registration is up to date. All of the insurance providers have arrangements whereby individual practitioners with low levels of earnings can obtain cover at a reduced cost. This varies from time to time and the current rates need to be sought from individual societies.

Recommended reading

Ellis N. *Employing staff*, 5th edn. London: BMJ Publishing Group, 1994.
Ellis N. *Making sense of general practice* Oxford: Radcliffe Medical Press, 1994.
Ellis N, Chisholm J. *Making sense of the Red Book*. Oxford: Radcliffe Medical Press, 1993.
Ellis N, Stanton A. *Making sense of partnerships*. Oxford: Radcliffe Medical Press, 1995.
Smith R. *The structure of general practice finance*. Frome: Publishing Initiatives Books, 1996.

5: Making the partnership work

The contractual obligation to provide 24 hour care for 365 days in every year will always tend to ensure that doctors have to find methods of working together. The way in which this is done for most is by partnership arrangements or by working together in practices. The NHS Terms of Service recognise this and have actively encouraged group practice formation financially in the recent past. The current contract has several aspects of pay which are practice- or partnership-based, such as cervical cytology target payments.

The creation of a happy and successful working relationship is not necessarily easy, and dysfunctional arrangements inevitably cause misery to the individuals and inhibit the delivery of good patient services. Professional relationships are as complex as marriages and the usual marriage counselling advice of listening to each other, considering each other's feelings and the need to work positively at making it successful, is very appropriate.

Are all practices inevitably partnerships?

The short answer to this question is no. Two or more doctors can choose to practice together in a grouped arrangement but this can only be said to be a partnership if there is a merging of some or all aspects of work and remuneration. Not all individuals find it easy to make the necessary compromises for true partnership but can find economies of scale through common operation of premises, equipment, and staff. Such an arrangement could still be called a group practice.

Partnership involves a degree of common responsibility for the delivery of services and has a status in law. It is important from the taxation point of view when a partnership is assessed as a complete unit. The 1996 taxation collection changes now determine that each partner is individually responsible for his or her personal tax payment while remaining subject to a global assessment.

The size of a partnership can be of any number more than one and can operate from more than one site. Making good relationships with many others in a large group is more complex and demands greater efforts at internal communication. A larger size partnership may be helped by a diversity of views and the availability of other members as mediators or negotiators.

Partnership agreements

It is always recommended that partnerships should have a legal agreement which is current. As a minimum this should specify the basis of joint working and the ownership and acquisition of the practice, its premises and equipment. It will definitely state the detail of the financial structure of the practice by determining how income has to be pooled and the profits divided. There is much more to making a happy partnership than this formal arrangement.

Cornerstones of happy partnerships

- Honesty and integrity
- Openness
- Understanding
- Equality
- Shared common objectives
- Shared loyalty to the organisation

Unfortunately it is often the absence of these features which is more easily identified and the encouragement of their adoption is much more difficult. A common mistake is to put too much weight and expectation on simple conformity. It is better to take a broad view, accepting and valuing each individual's attitude and knowledge as one of the features making for a successful relationship.

The need for honesty, integrity, and openness within a partnership needs little amplification. The facility for each member to have his or her views expressed and known to the others will not immediately solve every difficulty but will allow problem solving and planning to start from a realistic base. It is better that each member of a partnership makes known their personal discontents. This can lead on to argument, but that is usually less damaging in the longer term than simmering discontent. Understanding follows from this and provides a basis for making realistic levels of compromise which are always part of partnerships.

Equity, equality, and parity

These terms are not synonymous and need careful separation. Equity implies a commonly held view of fairness which can vary from time to time. It could well be fair that for a short time a new partner was receiving a smaller share or a partner nearer retirement received a smaller share in return for a reduced commitment.

Equality within a partnership can make relationships smoother and more effective but the search for absolute equality can be destructive. Reasonable levels of compromise are needed to allow for differing expertise, specialist roles, health, and attitudes. For example, the rigid adherence to the delivery of exactly the same number of consultations can be unrealistic if one partner is carrying all the load of minor surgery in the practice. Equality is also about having an equal share in the process of decision making.

Parity of income alone will avoid many conflicts but without a shared wish to make a practice successful, both in terms of patient care and professional and personal satisfaction, there is little likelihood of a happy partnership. The shared development of objectives and team working has to be deliberately encouraged by discussion and meeting.

The senior partner

Within partnerships there has often been a degree of apparent importance or even real power associated with all degrees of seniority. It was assumed that the senior partner would or should actively manage the practice and the other partners, and have a more significant say in decision making than others. By virtue of time and experience senior partners have a great deal of valuable knowledge and experience to bring to partnership activity.

Despite this, it is necessary and realistic to question the assumption of a senior partner's power both in the interests of that person and for the partnership as a whole. It also has to be considered in the context of the practice management arrangements which are discussed in a subsequent chapter. Not every member of a partnership will be equally interested or equipped to take a major role in management, in the same way that other individual members may not have equal knowledge or interest in training or diabetic care. It is therefore logical within a partnership for any work undertaken by partners to be done by the one with most interest in any particular field.

Managing partner or senior partner

One individual within a partnership will have to take a lead on management and organisation matters. This then leads to a concept of the "Managing Partner", who may be the senior but is not inevitably so. This will involve that person taking a greater interest and spending more time on the detail of practice management arrangements, with due allowance made for this by the others.

In some partnerships there may be no individual with such an interest or even several, in which case some arrangement of, say, yearly rotation of the managing partner role can be a solution. This can also be justified by the need to train in organisational skills. If such a rotation is adopted there is a danger that a partners may be forced to undertake more management than they wish, which results in less than adequate outcome and the neglect of problems or inadequate staff supervision, which has to be guarded against.

Making decisions

In a close relationship such as a partnership, the majority of decisions should be reached by consensus and agreement. If the pace is forced by voting and imposition, then the potential for discord arises. This does not mean that a single individual can always exercise a veto. The process of the group overruling one member should be approached cautiously and slowly.

Partnership agreements will usually specify the senior partner as having a casting vote in case of dispute and an even split of opinions. There is no reason why this cannot be assigned to the relevant managing partner if necessary and so specified in the agreement. In reality, any partnership decision taken on the basis of a casting vote is likely to be destructive to harmonious relationships and can dangerously reinforce differences of opinion. Autocratic senior partners making rapid forced decisions or exercising a veto are the cause of a large number of partnership disputes.

The spokesperson

Practice organisations are increasingly complex, both clinically and administratively, and there will be a need for a figurehead or spokesperson in many situations. This can vary in importance from making a presentation at a receptionist's retirement to answering questions from the local press. This obligation is likely to fall on the managing partner, whether senior or not, but can sometimes be assigned as a specific role separately to another member of the partnership. Again individual partners are likely to have different skills and aptitudes in this respect. The well-briefed, confident, forceful spokesperson, whether dealing with an application for an improvement grant with the health authority or a complaint by the Community Health Council, is more likely to produce an acceptable outcome than a diffident, reluctant practice representative.

It follows from the above that the terms of both senior and junior partner should not necessarily have particular roles ascribed to them. It is not reasonable to expect the newest arrived partner in the last year or two to have the same extent of knowledge as those more senior. Additionally, it is insulting to assume that a partner of many years' standing who happens to be younger is anything other than equal and to do otherwise will markedly degrade the partnership relationship.

Informal meeting and communication

There is no acceptable substitute for the face-to-face contact of partners which needs to be both formal and informal. Very large partnerships, less than full-time partners, and those working on split sites have particular difficulties in this respect and should consider the development of specific mechanisms to facilitate informal contact. The ideal will always be protected time free of interruptions every day at a fixed time. This may be the coffee break or just before starting the morning's work; it can be an informal lunch or sandwich together. The fact that inevitably not all partners will be able to be present on every day need not detract from the usefulness.

The prime focus of these meetings is the exchange of clinical information, such as the handover of individual patients' care. They have a major educational and support role in obtaining advice from others on clinical management. All partners need to keep abreast of the latest management of clinical problems and older partners in particular usually prefer not to have to turn to the books and can admit their ignorance more easily in such informal meetings. New partners and registrars can gain additional information equally. The secondary role of such meetings is the day-by-day updating exemplified by information as to staff absences or roster changes. Minor administrative problems, especially of an urgent nature, which are not likely to be contentious can be dealt with expeditiously at this time if the partnership has not delegated that sort of decision making to the manager or a specified partner. Such informal gatherings are not and should not be the time for major decision making or policy development. They can usefully and sensibly determine the agenda for the next business meeting.

Practice business meetings

It is easy to understand why these can be seen as a boring chore. They remain essential because all practices have within themselves the capability of producing significant partnership income which can be optimised by controlling and planning both activity and expenditure. The meeting process can be expedited by formalities which can ease the organisation, facilitate a useful outcome, and minimise time wasting.

Criteria for effective business meetings

- Timing
- Preparation
- Agenda
- Chairmanship
- Action lists and minutes

Timing

There are several important aspects of timing which are probably relevant to the organisation of any meeting. The first must be the selection of a time which is most convenient to all the participants so that usually all partners are present. This may best be done perhaps by a working lunch type of arrangement, or inconvenience can be minimised by some form of rotation as to which day of the week, but whatever system is used each partner should clearly understand the arrangements and have advance warning sufficient to modify rosters and commitments as necessary.

Part of this process must be deciding the length of a meeting. A maximum should normally be about two hours because after this concentration falls off and it is unlikely to be feasible to isolate more time than this on a regular basis. Regular business meetings are necessary but the amount of business will vary. A reasonable maximum could be a monthly meeting. A pattern of two hour meetings over a working lunch for say ten months of the year will probably be more than adequate for most, providing some other principles are followed.

Meeting preparation

Any meeting will progress much more speedily and efficiently if there is advance preparation, with, first, an agenda and, secondly, relevant information. A discussion as to staff salaries, for example, will always need reminders of the current situation and calculations of the probable costs of change. Decisions on refurbishment are unlikely to be meaningful without plans or quotations obtained in advance. If such an agenda and relevant information is circulated in advance it will facilitate the best use of partner time. These tasks should normally be undertaken by the manager with some guidance from the managing or other relevant partners.

An outline agenda

- Outcomes from the last meeting
- Regular reports – Finance
  – Staffing issues
  – Complaints
- Items for decision
- Items for information

In a small organisation the preparation of minutes can be burdensome. As an alternative the preparation of an action list is a useful tool. This should list briefly the major decisions taken and a name alongside each person responsible for their implementation who will report back to the next meeting. Using an action list alone can sometimes miss agreements of the more philosophical type and therefore lead to a need for amplification. To avoid difficulties in future it is probably best practice to keep minutes and prepare action lists and this should be a task delegated to the practice manager.

Do we need a meeting chairman?

The major role of an efficient chairman is to ensure that the meeting is well conducted and has a useful outcome. The first part of this will be timekeeping and the accompanying process of encouraging, or alternatively positively deciding to postpone, the taking of decisions. The next is to make sure that everyone present has had an appropriate opportunity to express their opinions. As a generality a chaired meeting will make the best use of available time.

Other partnership meetings

So far this text has concentrated on the business type of activity within the practice. It is not always possible or desirable to separate this clearly from clinical activity. In the context of making partnerships work, additional clinical focused meetings are just as important. These can have a main focus around clinical audit, preparation of clinical guidelines, development of practice formularies, and general educational purposes. Such meetings can also usefully meet Continuing Medical Education criteria if appropriately approved. All will help with the general cohesiveness of the partnership and feed into or from the business aspect.

Time-out and away days

Very difficult problems or complex patterns of problems may well need more time and resources than normal to solve. Arranging a time-out or away day can be helpful. Usually locums have to be found but this can be minimal, say for a Saturday, and a venue away from the usual pressures and telephones. The value can sometimes be enhanced by the use of a skilled facilitator who can guide the process. Suitable names can often be found through local contacts, the health authority, and professional organisations.

It is difficult to undertake such a process without some significant expenditure but the experience of many is that the process is extremely useful. Sometimes the pharmaceutical representatives can help and funds can be obtained from health authorities to assist team building. Such activities are also justified activity under the management arrangements for fundholding.

The duty of care

For a partnership to function each member has to have a degree of consideration of each other. All human beings have personal habits, preferences, and opinions to which they are entitled. Being a partner does not mean that they have to be stifled unreasonably and often they are best expressed even if that is sometimes uncomfortable. The ability to listen and tolerate marks out the human form and is to be encouraged in partnerships.

Part of this is also the need to detect, understand, and help each other in times of distress. Partners should recognise signs of stress, illness and unhappiness and do all that they can to mutually support and care. The opportunity of a sympathetic hearing may be enough, but may include guidance to access outside help. This must also extend into the most difficult areas of alcohol and drug abuse. The temptation to ignore or collude may be temporarily convenient but is more damaging in the long term. The partnership environment which does not accept and understand this need is not likely to be either successful or happy. Individual's religious and ethical beliefs must always be respected.

In these days of continuing escalation of complaints and litigation most partnerships will see from time to time one of their members under particular pressure for this reason. All are fallible and can find themselves at the receiving end of both justified and unjustified actions. Sympathetic understanding and listening can be tremendously supportive and help to prevent serious harm.

The social relationship

There is no harm in a partnership being entirely a business relationship. In some practices, because of familial or marital commitments, the personal and professional dimensions are inextricably mixed and cannot be divided. The majority of doctors do see the need to have, and use, personal time away from the pressure and stresses of work and this is not always easy when socialising with partners.

Many partnerships have found that the undue presence and influence of non-participants distorts practice relationships. Whilst not wishing to avoid all social contact it may well be best to regard the practice business as something quite distinct and separate from partners' private lives and personal relationships. The additional complication of partnerships employing the relatives of partners is full of potential for conflict and should not be commenced without fully considering all the possible consequences.

From time to time within partnerships and their staff emotional entanglements will occur. If the individuals concerned do not have marital commitments then there is less likelihood of upset. Conversely, major upsets will occur and should be considered carefully. It is particularly problematic if a relationship develops between a partner and an employee, as accusations of sexual harassment can easily arise. The best advice that can be given is to ensure that there is the maximum of separation between the practice and social activity.

Helping the troubled partnership

Inevitably some partnerships develop situations where relationships are deteriorating or stressed. It is usually in all the partners' interests and those of the patients and dependent staff to try to resolve conflicts and improve relationships. The LMC Secretaries have a particular counselling role to play in these situations and will help. If the particular individual Secretary is thought to be too close to a practice or an individual, then they can usually find an alternative acceptable to the partners.

Additionally, the Industrial Relations Officers or the BMA can offer help.

The officers of the health authority have an interest in continuing practice happiness and viability. They are a further source of help and counselling. Organising time, as in the time-out arrangements described above, can be helpful, as can some of the more formal team building courses and exercises.

Recommended reading

Adair J. *Effective team building*. London: Gower, 1986.

Ellis N, Stanton A. *Making sense of partnerships*. Oxford: Radcliffe Medical Press, 1995.

Lock, S (ed). *Organising a practice*. London: BMA, 1983.

Pringle M, Bilku J, Dornan M, Head S. *Managing change in primary care*. Oxford: Radcliffe Medical Press, 1991.

6: Practice management structure

Why worry?

Practices have become large and complex organisations which fail in their core functions if they are not organised and managed. Simultaneously that process can in itself be costly and unnecessarily bureaucratic without intelligent guidance. The way in which a practice is best managed with the most appropriate structure and staff depends on two variables, the first of which is the size of the practice and the second is the extent to which doctors are prepared to permit and encourage delegation to employed staff.

For any organisation to function, whether large and complex or small and simple, it must have some purpose to its existence. This purpose and function needs to be understood and accepted by all involved. Two objectives will dominate any practice organisation, and these are providing for the needs of patients and providing a living for the partners.

The components of management

The main components

- Leadership
- Management
- Administration

These three components are fundamentally different but have large overlaps, and it may be difficult to separate them totally.

Leadership

The leadership role

- Developing a vision
- Setting the objectives
- Assigning the tasks
- Teaching
- Encouraging cohesion and common endeavour

Using current jargon, leadership functions can be expressed as visioning, organisational philosophy, and strategic direction. Inevitably the major part of this must come from the doctors in their role in service delivery, knowledge of practice and their position as owners of the business. In a partnership these perspectives and objectives need to be agreed or the organisation will be strained by pulling in opposite directions.

Management

What is management?

- Converting the vision to action
- The accumulation and organisation of information
- Process organisation
- Organising training
- Monitoring results
- Controlling the budget

These are functions which can be performed by doctors alone, and frequently are in the single-handed practice. They are time-intensive activities additionally needing education in financial skills and personnel management which are not usually part of the general practitioner's training. Done well, they can be economical or even profit-creating, done badly they will interfere with the ability of the doctor to do what he or she is trained for – medical care. This is the justification for the development of the Practice Manager, but this can only work where doctors are prepared to delegate and cooperate.

Administration

What is administration?

- Clerical process work
- Recording
- Completing documentation
- Collecting data

Components of administration are found in the work of all team members, including doctors and managers, and are not always avoidable. They should be delegated wherever possible to minimise the waste of expensive staff time. With the complex nature of the practitioner's remuneration structure, the accurate honest completion of documentation is vital for practice profitability. An efficient administration will ensure income and minimise loss in a way that can be partially self-financing.

Delegation and monitoring

The development of the concept of practice management in general practice is very variable and much confused. It has been characterised often by a reluctance of doctors to delegate work and empower their employees. This is somewhat understandable as many have entered general practice because of the cherished facility of being able to control their own affairs and work. It does, however, contrast with the clinical aspects of their work, where for many years doctors have been increasingly delegating tasks to nurses and other clinical staff.

Feeling comfortable with delegation

- Understand the employee's knowledge and skills
- Arrange appropriate training
- Monitor the delegated process
- Check the outcome

These simple rules should be applied with a light touch and a trusting approach and are equally applicable to clinical delegation.

What should the manager do?

It is possible to answer this question with a long list of tasks but it is probably better to consider the necessary range of skills and knowledge, under which headings the particular tasks can be allocated. The skill range will be universal throughout practices, whatever their size, and needs to be provided whether by dedicated managers or by practitioners themselves. Tasks under these headings can be undertaken by the manager or assigned to a formal deputy or some other member of staff who will take responsibility for their delivery.

Key managerial roles

- Planning and organisation
- Financial monitoring and control
- Personnel management
- Communication and liaison
- Project management
- Resource management
- Fund management

Planning by managers can superficially sound like a process of controlling the doctors, when in this context it means organising and facilitating in a way that allows them to devote the maximum of their time to clinical duties. Usually doctors can earn more by spending their time on clinical activity or benefit by releasing time for recreational activity rather than spending their time on planning detail.

The practical aspects of financial monitoring and control are vital to the business health of any practice and its profitability. The processes of budget setting, control, and bookkeeping are complex and time-consuming, involving copious paper work and should be delegated. The presentation of clear, concise financial information helps to elucidate many problems. Similarly staff recruitment, training, and discipline need detailed skills not owned by most practitioners and can be delegated.

Increasingly practices have to communicate at an organisational level with outside bodies, which is time-consuming yet frequently to their advantage. This, combined with the need to develop and operate in-house complaint systems, is easily delegated to an appropriately trained manager.

When decisions are taken by partners they need to be translated into detailed action. This is project management and is allied to the process of resource management which encompasses all the routines of ensuring that the practice is in full working order. Premises and equipment maintenance, supplies, and routine staff organisation are distractions to clinical practice.

Fund management

This demands an extra range of skills more fully developed than in much of traditional practice activity.

Management tasks specific to fundholding

- Budget negotiation
- Contract development
- Contract negotiation
- Contract monitoring
- Specified computerised accounting
- Forward projection and estimating

These add a major slice of work to the management activity of the practice and need to be closely interrelated to the health needs of the practice population and the doctor's clinical actions. Their size and complexity mean that a different style of management is needed where it will be necessary to employ a dedicated person who has a higher level of intellectual capability and training. Individual practices have approached this in different ways, many originally opting for an additional dedicated fund manager. As the scope of fundholding has extended, it is becoming apparent that a more successful pattern is to have a single overall practice manager covering all aspects with a very advanced level of training and education. This person can then be supported by assistants and clerical staff with clear lines of responsibility and levels of delegation.

How are managers trained?

The first practice managers were home-grown by gradually extending the role of a currently employed member of staff. Without a great deal of training, both internal and external to the practice, this can lead to a very narrow perspective and skill range. It is also frequently accompanied by a reluctance by doctors to be totally open and see the manager as a valued and trusted colleague. A process of adding increasing amounts of responsibility and duties on an existing employee produces someone who can be very competent in a limited range of activities but be lacking in vision. This can also be associated with a resistance to change and a slow pace of learning. Management demands a wide range of skills and an ability to understand practice activity both in the context of partner's investment and profitability alongside the complex activities of the wider health service

The consequence of this is the development of specific practice management training.

Practice management training

- AMSPAR – Certificate and Diploma in Practice Management
- Association of Managers in General Practice Diploma
- Health service graduate management training schemes
- Higher degree in business management at MBA level
- Institute of Health Service Management membership

All the qualifications detailed in the Box need to be based around the university graduate level and can usefully be added on to the business studies type of degree course. In many aspects management is a generic skill capable of transfer between businesses of many different forms. Therefore individuals who have undergone training or gained experience in other spheres can be good recruits but obviously need more induction into the specifics of practice. The assumption that anyone who is mainly adept at numerical work, perhaps characterised by ex-bankers, is therefore suitable managerial material disregards the much wider range of knowledge and ability needed.

Whatever the original discipline or training the continuing education of managerial staff must not be neglected. They need to be encouraged to take part in education with their own peer groups, take advantage of all education offers and continue to read widely. Inevitably this will also mean some degree of turnover of staff, as a period spent as a practice manager is increasingly viewed as necessary to health service management career development. The intermittent infusion of new managers into practices has a positive quality of continually increasing skills.

Maximising the value of a manager

Management is a skill with a real contribution to make to efficient profitable practice operation. This means that much thought should be given to the exact job description and type of person needed prior to appointment. Doctors need to facilitate and guide this in a manner which suits their own needs. This will always involve the setting of clear objectives and a realistic level of delegation and trust.

Principal elements of the managerial job description

- Office organisation
- Staff recruitment, training, and supervision
- Staff personal review
- Managing income claiming and collection
- Financial recording, budget creation, and monitoring.
- Computer supervision
- Purchase management
- Receiving and investigating complaints
- Information collection and manipulation
- Business planning and project development
- Fund management

These are only broad categories which will need to be described in detail as they will vary between practices. The partners do not need large amounts of detailed information in a well organised system but they do need to monitor management activity and have realistic checking mechanisms. This will always include ready access to all information and a recognised regular reporting process both verbal and written. Practical measures such as countersignature and specified financial levels of delegation will be part of the procedures.

It can be difficult to accept change or innovation arising from initiatives from managers. Their value will be increased by rational attentive consideration of their suggestions whilst not committing to blind acceptance. A manager who is not made to feel a valued member of the whole team with a real contribution to make is unlikely to earn his or her keep. Equally, unless a manager has full open access to all the information on the practice, he or she will be operating in an expensive wasteful vacuum. The effective manager will need to take part in almost all partnership meetings, both to provide information, understand the objectives, and receive instructions.

Routine managerial reporting

- Current accounts including cash flow
- Staff matters – absence
  – training
  – recruitment
- Exceptional equipment and maintenance problems
- Progress on current activity and targets

Too small to need a manager?

Small practices have a problem in running their business alone without any managerial help. Inevitably precious time is lost from remunerative clinical work or from leisure time undertaking tasks which doctors do not enjoy and therefore perform poorly. As a minimum, the principle must be to delegate whenever possible and to develop systematic approaches to essential tasks. Individual employees work roles need to be optimised so that routine administrative tasks are completed alongside other activity and this is regularly checked.

There is also scope, which is already seen in fund management, to share staff on a variety of arrangements. With good professionals, confidentiality should be assured and specific allocation of hours can be negotiated and funded by a number of practices. To some extent the accountancy practices which have specialised in general practice are beginning to offer this type of service on a contracted basis, which may have attractions to some despite the concept being rather poorly developed. Additionally, use can be made of commercial bookkeeping services, which can be helpful, cheaper than accountants, and minimise distraction from clinical services.

Recommended reading

Applebee K, Morgan S, Sawyer B (eds). *Croner's general practice manager.* London: Croner Publications, 1995.

Drury M, Hobden-Clarke L. *The practice manager* 3rd edn. Oxford: Radcliffe Medical Press, 1994.

Henry S, Pickersgill D (eds). *Making sense of fundholding.* Oxford: Radcliffe Medical Press, 1995.

Pirie A, Kelly M (eds). *Fund holding, a practice guide.* Oxford: Radcliffe Medical Press, 1992.

Pritchard P, Low K, Whalen M. *Management in general practice.* Oxford: Oxford Medical Publications, 1984.

Williams S. *Making best practice better.* Frome: Publishing Initiatives Books, 1994.

7: Primary care skill mix and making the team work

Modern primary care and general practice needs a wide range of skills and knowledge, and therefore the ability of any individual doctor to be fully competent and operate entirely independently is limited. The need for nursing skills has been recognised for many years and there is an increasing involvement of other professionals within the team. The cooperative delivery of appropriate and effective primary health care demands the recognition of the need to work in teams, which in itself places demands on those involved.

The classic primary health care team

- General practitioners
- Community (district) nurses
- Health visitors
- Midwife
- Administrative staff

A single team comprising the mix of members shown, working together from one base jointly providing care for the practice population, has gained general acceptance in general practice circles. That acceptance has not been universal, however, for several reasons, one of the most significant being the objections of the nursing profession. There has been anxiety that this was some form of empire building by doctors, relegating nurses to a doctor's handmaiden position and failing to recognise their professionalism and value their contribution to the management and planning aspects of primary care. There have also been problems as to the leadership role, with nurses frequently advocating a principle that team working, by its nature, implies denying any role for the doctor to provide strategic direction. There has therefore been pressure to try to deliver the range of nursing services on a separate geographical zoned basis from separate premises. More recently, however, the Primary Health Care Team concept is gaining greater acceptance.

Whilst this structure is the core, the nature of its work is being continuously altered by changing medical knowledge and practice. An example of this is the changing nature and style of midwifery practice. Medical practitioners are no longer generally involved in large amounts of *intra partum* care and the practice midwife has tended almost to become an independent practitioner, providing services from the practice base and spending much time acting as the practice liaison with the hospital maternity unit.

Primary care nursing roles

Practice nurses have developed separately from community nurses, with their own distinct training and work role. It is therefore useful to consider the range of nursing involved in primary care and how that relates to general practice.

Primary care nursing disciplines

- Practice nursing
- Community nursing
- Health visiting
- Midwifery
- Community psychiatric nursing
- Learning disability nursing
- Speciality advisory nursing – diabetes
  - – stoma services
  - – continence
  - – palliative care (Macmillan nursing)
  - – respiratory care
  - – etc.
- Nurse practitioners

Inevitably the list given will not be complete, and different names are used in various parts of the health service. Additionally, there is further complexity produced by different levels of grading and or qualification within each branch and the extent to which individuals are hospital outreach workers or entirely community-based. Some function entirely by direct application of nursing skills to patients and others function partly or wholly as advisers to other nurses.

The complexities of the number of nurses with wide ranging and different skills supplying services to the practice population has led some to make a division between the core Primary Health Care Team and the Extended Team, the separation being made on the basis of those who are almost totally individually practice-based, with practice-delivered services, and those with more limited contact.

Nurse practitioners

This concept of a nurse with an advanced level of nurse training and experience allowing a greater degree of independent practice, particularly in the areas of examination and investigation, diagnosis, and treatment initiation, is well recognised throughout much of the world. The role has developed in a number of different forms, sometimes working alongside doctors or alternatively at a distance. Some are trained at an advanced level across a range of medical activity and others in depth in a more limited field.

In the United Kingdom this concept is only just gaining ground at the present time, despite the fact that midwives have operated in this way for some time. As this role develops it becomes a clear example of skill mix change or skill dilution where nurses are partially taking on tasks and roles which previously would have been regarded as medical. Nurse practitioners therefore can relieve doctors of a significant portion of their work, thus releasing them for other activities.

Other members of the team

Other workers are seen as integral to the Primary Health Care Team because they provide a range of skills that are very useful and necessary for patient care and are not owned by other team members. They usually operate within the team centre, cooperating with others. Doubtless as time progresses further skills will be added, producing even more complexity to the team organisation.

Team members with additional clinical skills

- Counsellors
- Physiotherapists
- Dieticians
- Chiropodists

The managerial and administrative team

It is easy to neglect the vital role of this part of the Primary Health Care Team. They facilitate all the activity and release clinicians from unnecessary administrative tasks. To do this well they need to understand and share the objectives of the team and be involved in joint education and training.

Creating team spirit

One common feature of all team members, whether doctors, partners, employed, attached or associated, is their obligation to serve the practice patients in a particular locality. The continual emphasis in everything that is done should be on the value to patients. This motivation helps to overcome concepts of professional superiority and boundaries. It emphasises the interdependence of skills and abilities as rarely will one member alone be able to satisfy any individual patient's total needs over a period of time.

Criteria for effective team working

- Well-trained individuals with appropriate skills
- Understanding of individuals' limitations and professional boundaries
- Willingness to compromise
- Shared desire to communicate
- Shared common objectives
- Shared commitment to the service users and practice population

A team will never work if the individuals within it do not know and understand the role and abilities of each member, including their limitations, whether due to education, inexperience or professional boundaries. Team working for primary care has a major advantage in that it is relatively easy for all to agree that the purpose of its existence is to provide for the health needs of a defined population group, the practice population. The majority of health workers have made a commitment to patient care from the moment they start training and this can be built upon.

Communication

Most organisations, including practice teams, need to have an understanding of the dynamics of interpersonal relationships. This extends from the courtesies of greetings and politeness to the style of addressing each other. The use of first names in our society is increasing, yet if the doctor always expects the use of his or her title while addressing subordinates by their first name or surname, it will be seen as offensively patronising. Politeness in communication does not interfere with the exertion of authority. The expression and communication of thanks, combined with polite and non-intrusive interest in other team members, is usually repaid in better working relationships.

Communication within the team

- Informal
- Formal
- Educational
- Social

The very best communications occur when two people meet face to face on an equal basis, willing to listen and to be heard. This is the most informal communication; it is very effective and actually facilitates the building of mutual respect which allows other communications to develop. A telephone conversation between two people who have never met will never be as valuable as that between individuals who already know each other. Similarly written messages have an enhanced value between known correspondents.

Inevitably it is going to be harder work where team members are not based in the same premises or share the same facilities. The open door inviting access and the shared coffee break or shared common room might seem to be an invitation to waste time but actually is a good investment of time in team building. Doctors are frequently in danger of believing that their time is more important than that of any other team member, but a few moments spent in going to see another member in their room is far preferable for team dynamics than a demand that others slavishly attend on the doctor. Communicating is always a two-way process of listening and speaking.

Team meetings

As teams become larger, the logistics of formal meetings become more difficult. They tend to be more formalised and lacking in spontaneity, and individual practices may not have an adequate space to use. Despite this, the occasional event will help individuals to see their role in a larger perspective.

For routine purposes smaller group meetings of representatives or sections of the organisation can be substituted.

Simplistic effective motivation

- Good working environment
- Appropriate equipment
- Uniforms and badges

The provision of a good working environment will not in itself produce good team working, but only rarely will the pressure of adversity weld the team together. Personal and group pride gives rise to enthusiasm and is encouraged by bright, clean, and appropriate facilities. Equipment does not need to be over-provided but it does need to be in good working order. All staff, whether doctors, administrative or clinical, feel much more valued and give their best with decent tools, and certainly do not happily spend their working days in an environment less cheerful than their own homes.

Creating a corporate identity

The provision and use of uniforms encourages a corporate feeling and pride in the organisation. It is not necessarily expensive and many specialist suppliers are available. Name badges stating name, job and organisation title are simple but helpful. For attached or linked staff employed by others, direct practice control over these matters is not possible but the encouragement of use of their own and possibly additional badges can be helpful.

Training

Education is very important for the development of team working. The roles and responsibilities of the team members and the corporate group are the basics. When each team member knows the extent and limitations of each other's skills and training it becomes easier to accept whoever leads in a particular situation. The process of being jointly educated can produce enormous benefits. Educational efforts can and should be made to develop team working.

Ideally all the team members should have a protected time away from the practice together for this purpose. This is unlikely to be feasible in any substantial way but groups of team members, usually from various disciplines, can be released to an educational environment where they can be taught interpersonal skills and practice theoretical and practical problem solving and develop ideas to return to the whole team.

Communication tips

Formal methods of communication and interrelation have a significant part in facilitating team work. Specific message books and internal memos are all useful providing that there is a will to make them work. Their value can be further enhanced by colour coding and specified collection points and timed collection and delivery.

A very important time for formal communication is when practice objectives and plans are being developed or agreed. Without some degree of ownership of the process of development the team will not readily cooperate in their execution. This is when meetings do become essential.

In large organisations there is a useful place for written internal memos or even occasional newsletters. Notice boards in the staff areas are also useful aids to ensure communication. The combination of these methods will ensure that no individual can claim not to have been told of matters of importance.

Social interaction

Some degree of social interaction within a team will always occur and can help team work. Too great a pressure to encourage individuals to socialise can be counter-productive and most do not need to be reminded of the pressures of work in their private time. Despite this, the effort of organising and financing the occasional event such as the Christmas Party is useful for morale. The introduction of spouses of team members in such a function often helps to smooth communication and lessen insecurities in what can sometimes seem to be a very hierarchical structure.

Practitioners can usefully help these things along with an investment of time and finance which will be amply repaid. The provision by practices of simple refreshments for breaks and working lunches will not encourage time wasting but will simplify the task of ensuring that individuals relate sufficiently to function together.

Monitoring the team

As in most things in life, some anticipatory care is better than repairing a damaged machine. However, in all organisations over a period of time there will be some staff turnover, new tasks will be introduced and others made obsolete. Individuals will change in their personality or attitude whether due to external influences or not. This will have effects on team relationships.

Danger signs of team malfunction

- Interpersonal disputes
- Repeated errors
- Increasing complaints
- Timekeeping problems
- Absenteeism
- Increased sickness absence

An increasing level of any or all of the danger signs listed is extremely significant and demands careful attention and action to investigate and correct. Time spent at an early stage by a manager or the doctor will usually not be wasted. The nature of the necessary correction will vary but will always involve assessing the state of communications within the practice and a degree of education or re-training.

When the inevitable staff changes occur, care and courtesy in the process by formal thanks and presentations will be encouraging to the remainder of the team. Simultaneously, a final private interview can often be very revealing and provide useful intelligence on staff morale and opinion.

Recommended reading

Adair J. *Effective team building.* London: Gower, 1986.

Anon. *Buying community nursing, a guide for GPs.* London: Royal College of Nursing, 1993.

Anon. *Nursing in primary health care – new world, new opportunities.* Leeds: NHS Management Executive, 1993.

Bowling A, Stilwell B, (eds). *The nurse in family practice. Practice nurses and nurse practitioners in family health care.* London: Scutari Press, 1988.

Ellis N. *Employing staff,* 5th edn. London: BMJ Publishing Group, 1994.

Marsh G. *Efficient care in general practice.* Oxford: Oxford University Press, 1992.

Pearson A, Vaughan B. *Nursing models from practice.* Portsmouth: Heinemann Nursing, 1990.

8: Practice housekeeping

This chapter is intended to guide practitioners on the organisation of some simple but significant aspects of practice management. There are two immediate advantages of good housekeeping: every practice spends substantial amounts on routine activities in this area, which if managed effectively can minimise cost and maximise profitability; secondly, it is important not to divert expensively acquired medical or any other staff time needlessly coping with problems or shortages which could have been anticipated.

Additionally covered under this heading are the obligations created by the need of the practice to act as an employer and by having members of the public on the premises. These obligations are shared by all forms of business enterprises whether large or small. This involves some knowledge of a number of statutory requirements, the enforcement of which is backed by legal penalties.

Legislation and regulations

The regulatory framework can appear to be both tedious and unnecessary in the context of general practice, but there is potential risk in ignoring the possible occurrence of the unexpected. All the necessary actions which follow can be delegated to a manager, but they do potentially carry significant expenditure implications.

Legislative and regulatory obligations

- Public liability and associated insurance
- Employee protection and associated insurance
- Data protection and information technology security
- Fire safety
- Health and safety
- Waste management

Public and employee liability

The need for general public and employee liability arises from the chance of accidents happening on the practice premises or where the practitioners and their staff are functioning, which is not of a direct clinical practice nature. In general this means that there is an obligation to ensure safety, varying from ensuring the ceiling will not collapse to dealing with the presence of loose carpeting on staircases. Insurance to cover these risks is often sold as part of a package covering other things such as fire and theft. Insurers have the right to expect a certain level of diligence on the part of their customers and are increasingly offering both written advice and the availability of inspection as part of their contracts. Current relevant insurance certificates have to be displayed to staff and the public.

Information technology security

Doctors using computer systems are usually aware of the data protection legislation which mandates and controls the use and access to the system. This will be dealt with more fully elsewhere in the text. There is a much less well-known obligation for the physical security of the equipment. The aim of this is to ensure that the data cannot be easily stolen along with the system. Copies of data held have to be stored separately and securely away from the hardware. The hardware itself should be physically secured so that it cannot easily be removed.

Fire safety

The risk of fire in any practice premises is probably quite small and centres around heating and electrical equipment. As premises and operations become more complex, these risks begin to increase. Additional problems concern means of escape and congestion, especially with regard to people who may have limitations on their mobility.

Elements of fire safety

- Prevention
- Fire alarms
- Means of escape
- Extinguishers

The prevention of fire must include the initial installation of safe equipment and its regular checking and maintenance. All new building needs to be approved from a fire safety point of view, both in its design and building standards, which is usually coordinated by designers and architects. The local fire services will undertake inspections and make recommendations on exits, escapes, alarms, and extinguishers. Automatic smoke and carbon monoxide detectors are readily available and should be used alongside manually activated alarms.

The fire service will advise on escape routines and help to organise appropriate staff training. It may not be mandatory to follow the advice given, but if ignored it may invalidate insurance cover. Most importantly, it is necessary to ensure that all staff are well trained in their personal role in the event of a fire.

Health and safety

Health and safety legislation is complex and extensive. It places obligations on employers and employees and has to be seen alongside various specialised regulations.

Regulatory principles

- Hazards should be anticipated
- Hazards should be made known to the workforce
- Systems to avoid hazards should be developed
- Necessary equipment for the handling of hazards should be available
- Staff should be trained on appropriate techniques by competent trainers
- Staff are mandated to follow approved practices

The most significant aspect of this for general practice is the understanding of what constitutes a hazard. Clinical staff easily recognise that damaged furniture could easily hurt themselves or a patient but may not so readily accept that there is a potential hazard in assisting patients to dress. The process of identifying hazards should be a joint exercise by managers and employees and can be assisted by various checklists, but these will generally only cover the commonest problems.

Identified hazards then need to be assessed as to whether it is possible to remove them totally and what action can be taken to minimise risk. All of this should be the responsibility of the manager who then has to develop responses, train staff in their use, and continuously monitor the whole process.

Waste management

Waste management is subject to regulation and approved procedures. This is discussed on p. 79.

Parallel issues

Whilst technically separate, there are a number of areas of regulation which are similar. The Control of Substances Hazardous to Health regulations cover the handling and storage of materials as diverse as domestic cleaning materials used on the premises to fixatives used in the preparation of cervical cytology slides. The principles to be followed are broadly similar.

The use of autoclaves presents special hazards of explosion and is covered by separate legislation. Insurers will also wish to specify routine inspection and certification as a prior condition to cover.

Similarly, insurers are insisting on evidence of routine regular examination of electrical equipment and wiring. Attention to their demands will ensure simultaneous legislative compliance. The area covered by these types of regulation extends on a regular basis and may have relevance. Modern noisy office equipment may exceed approved noise levels in the workplace and so on.

Purchasing

The potential for both wastage and economy in this area can have significant effects on practice profitability. Extreme levels of economy can also result in damage to the image and activity of the practice. Sensible levels of compromise should be developed. This can be exemplified by the regular purchase of stationery items where the slightly higher cost of coordinated quality items has a beneficial effect on the practice image. This does not detract from the process of seeking the most economical supplier.

Supplies and consumables

This is a major expense in operating any organisation where the absence of even quite small items can cause chaos. The corner shop can be used to obtain a quick supply of tissues but they are unlikely to stock auroscope bulbs. Therefore there needs to be some concept of the minimum stock to be held in the practice, of both continuously used items and occasional needs, balanced against the speed at which replacements can be delivered.

Medical equipment from specialist suppliers may take days to deliver but some items are available from myriad local competitive suppliers. The maintenance of a larger stock of some continuously used items can sometimes be justified if this allows advantageous financial terms. The prices obtained from regular suppliers can vary considerably over a period of time. Whatever compromise is decided, it will not work unless some individual is clearly given the responsibility and authority to check continuously and order as appropriate. Checking a variety of sources can show wide divergence on costs for many items.

It is easily forgotten that alternative suppliers are available for staple items. Electricity and gas can be bought from competing suppliers, as can telephone services. These contracts often need to be longer term but regular review can be remunerative.

Acquisition of major equipment items

When new major items are required there is a need to look at competing prices and methods of financing. It will be worth an opinion from the practice accountants as to the current most tax-efficient process and timing. It is possible to hire or lease many items and this may meet practice needs by minimising capital expenditure and extended credit terms can be on offer. There are many sorts of business development loans offered by the banks and all these methods can have different taxation consequences, as can the exact date of the transaction.

Maintenance

This can easily absorb a significant percentage of practice income and can be disproportionately upsetting to the cash flow situation. Sudden unexpected large costs are best avoided if at all possible. Some items can be anticipated, such as decorating, which means that a plan to phase this over a few years in equal amounts is possible. A dedicated budget for this can be developed.

In a similar way the routine need to repair and replace items of practice equipment, varying from chairs to stethoscopes, can be anticipated. Delayed repair and replacement often results in increased expenditure and the allocation of a budget for these items can ease their financial management. If desired such a budget can be enhanced sufficient to fund a rolling programme of replacement or minor improvement.

Additional thought can usefully be given to the durability of practice fittings and furnishing to minimise expenditure. For example, in some areas decoratively finished brickwork can be cheaper to maintain than painted walls; substantial fixed waiting room seating of the commercial types used in restaurants and public houses is usually more durable and not necessarily more expensive than ordinary domestic furniture.

Inventories and records

As premises become larger and more comprehensively equipped it is useful to keep a room inventory. This need only be a simple file which records the contents and their date of acquisition and the date of the last redecoration or upgrading. It will help the practice to anticipate expenditure and be very useful if any insurance claims have to be made for any reason.

Preferred providers of services

It is often quite difficult to obtain the reliable services of tradesmen in an emergency or for minor tasks. It is therefore sensible to develop a list of the preferred tradesmen with whom a long term relationship can be developed. Costs can be minimised by only calling on their services when a few items can be dealt with simultaneously, and is helped by a fault recording system.

Despite the foregoing, when more major projects are in hand, there needs to be a system of obtaining tenders to ensure that unexpected costs are not added and the most economical deal obtained. Practices need to understand and accept that where work is being done on premises in active use or out of hours this will increase the cost. The careful management of this work around holidays and so on in close discussion with the contractor can be financially advantageous.

Cleaning

Adequate reliable cleaning is essential for all practices and can minimise maintenance expenditure. Generally speaking, the direct employment of a known person is preferable to the use of contract services which have large overheads and less well-known staff. This also minimises problems arising from confidential material. On the other hand, even the most reliable cleaner will be absent on occasions and the work still needs to be done and temporary staff engaged and supervised. Contracted services can reduce the management and supervision task at the expense of having to develop systems of totally securing all confidential information.

Insurance

Checking the accounts of any practice will show that large sums of money are spent in this area. Insurance can be regarded as a commodity like other consumables, which means that shopping for competitive prices and questioning of potential insurers or their agents can minimise expenditure. This is not something that can be done casually, as inevitably the small print in policies can be vital. Equally the continued reliance on the dependable local agent may hide the fact that the practice is only offered the policy with the biggest margin for the agent and the disadvantages only become obvious when claims are made. Gaps in insurance cover are not unusual.

This is very much an area where the buyer needs to take care but economies and rationalisations are frequently worthwhile. Once again, there is a clear need for managerial control and interest.

Security

All aspects of security in a practice are significant and demand attention to reduce risk to individuals and to the practice assets. Many practices fail to develop proper approaches to personal security for doctors and staff, as significant events occur rarely. This is a false assumption, however, as violence in practices, both urban and rural, is an ever-increasing problem.

The risk needs recognition and demands the development of a policy including a continuing system of education aimed at prevention. Such a policy will include education on trying to recognise potential attackers, minimising reaction in stressful situations and calling for help at the earliest indication of a problem. All persons working alone with patients need a readily accessible unobtrusive alarm of the panic button type. Portable alarms of the noisy aerosol type to use outside of the practice premises are also useful.

The security of assets of the practice is best managed by a mixture of good procedures and physical restraint. The obvious first step is that when the surgery is open the receptionist staff must always know when a person enters the premises and when that person leaves. This can be a complex process but done efficiently it also helps the clinical process and appointment systems and works best when the premises have only one entrance.

Small items and especially prescription pads and written prescriptions should be kept unobtrusively at points where they are not easily reached by surgery attendees. Consideration should be given to closing and locking rooms or areas of the building not in use at a particular time. All removable items should be marked with the name of the practice in some indelible form.

The external security will almost certainly involve the need for an alarm system and suitable security lighting. A useful system is to have a written security checklist which details the checks to be made when securing the premises at the end of the day.

In all these areas of security, whether for personnel, property, or assets, police forces offer the free advice of crime prevention officers. They can also advise on self defence courses and the best defensive behaviour to avoid becoming a target when in the community.

Waste management

Practices produce large volumes of waste in their regular activity. It falls into several categories and its disposal can be controlled by legislation and medical protocols and even ethical considerations.

Categories of waste

- Clinical waste
- Used medical sharps
- Waste drugs and medications
- Confidential papers
- Routine domestic-type garbage

Each of these categories needs to be addressed separately and handled differently, the processes being determined by a need to protect both staff and the service users. Clinical waste is used dressings and materials which may have become contaminated by tissue and body fluids, including blood, but not sharps. It has to be separated and the method of disposal, including the temperature of incineration, defined. Such material in the practice has to be sealed and labelled for storage and isolated from staff and patient contact.

Separate arrangements are mandated for the collection and disposal of sharps and waste drugs. Some waste drugs have to be separated from their containers if glass, and waste aerosols must be kept separately. As with clinical waste, specialised contractors need to be used to comply with regulations and approved procedures. Doctors and staff need to be regularly reminded of their responsibilities in these areas.

Confidential waste

Practices produce large amounts of paper on which is written confidential and identifiable patient information. The volume can be quite large, especially if there is an active record management policy. The waste has to be separated from other domestic garbage and this can be done by having a separate marked or colour coded series of litter bins throughout the building. This waste can then be collected and shredded in house and then placed with normal domestic waste. Alternatively, it can be sealed and disposed of by specialist contractors who undertake to incinerate or pulp the material.

Recommended reading

Anon. *A step by step guide to COSSH Assessment.* London: Health and Safety Executive, 1993.

Anon. *Essentials of health and safety at work.* London: Health and Safety Executive, 1988.

Fry J, Scott K, Jeffree P. *Practice management compendium. Part 2: Organising the practice.* Norwelk: Kluwer Academic Press, 1990.

Moore R, Moore S. *Health and safety at work – guidance for general practitioners.* London: RCGP Practice Organisation Series, 1996.

Morgan D (ed.). *Code of practice for the safe use and disposal of sharps.* London: BMA, 1990.

9: Practice communications

One of the most important skills necessary for good general practice is the ability to communicate with patients. This is usually only considered within the consultation and ignores the use of a variety of communication methods. Outside of the privacy of the consultation and its confidentiality, many general health messages are worth spreading and reinforcing, as well as the regular notices of an administrative nature.

Effective communications almost inevitably involve an interchange, and attention to the return message can be valuable to the practice, giving useful insights as to the patients' opinions and understanding.

Rules of communication

- Clear messages
- Concisely expressed
- Readable language
- Attractive presentation.

Notices and notice boards

It is worth remembering that the reception and waiting areas are the shop window of the practice and help to attract and hold patients. The haphazard plastering of practice waiting rooms with numerous relevant and irrelevant notices and posters has been the limit of practice communications for some. If notices and posters are limited they can be very useful. They need to be readable, clearly expressing their message in a few words. Notice boards need to be limited to parts of the building, and if a number of areas are available each should have a dedicated task.

It is useful to have a single area for health education messages which covers a single topic and is changed frequently. The chosen topic could be in line with current national campaigns, with relevant leaflets available, or alternatively in line with more local priorities. One staff member should have this clearly specified as their responsibility and is an area of much interest to health visitors.

Another notice area might usefully be specified for administrative purposes and managed similarly to display information of relevance to current practice activity, such as opening hours, new services, and staff changes. Most practices find themselves inundated with requests to allow advertising in the surgery for myriad local needs, varying from jumble sales to adverts for lost pets. This can give rise to an untidy and uninformative clutter. To avoid the risk of offending individual patients, folders with transparent pockets can be made available for use in the waiting room for such advertisements.

Practice leaflets

There have always been anxieties as to the extent to which the production of a practice leaflet constitutes advertising, prohibited by medical ethics. The current view is that such a document is only unethical if it is distributed on an unsolicited basis and not confined to active or prospective patients of the practice. The provision of an attractive practice leaflet is a very useful tool to communicate both with new and existing patients. There is a conflict as to the amount of detail necessary, and unless controlled, a profusion of contents will make the document unreadable.

Minimum leaflet contents

- Names, sex, and age of the doctors
- Physical location of the practice
- Usual hours of service
- Arrangements for telephone contact
- Arrangements for out of hours services
- Details of the doctors' special interests
- Lists of services provided
- Mechanisms for making suggestions and complaints

A brief explicit leaflet which is attractively designed can present the basic detail quite economically. The information can be made more explicit by amplification of the detail and additional information. It can be helpful to list the names of all the team and explain their roles and training. If any training is undertaken in the practice on a regular basis, this needs explanation. The whole document can then be enlarged with the provision of guidance as to health promotion and self management of minor illness, including simple first aid.

Inevitably as the document grows from a leaflet towards a booklet, difficulties of readability and cost will arise. A good designer can help to present an individual attractive image by means of layout, order, emphasis, and colour. There are some publishing companies who specialise in this field. They can produce suitable leaflets free of charge with assistance by the practice in obtaining suitable advertising and revenue therefrom. This has to be handled with some discretion as the presence of advertisements in a practice leaflet can be interpreted by some patients as a positive recommendation with some consequent conflicts.

Newsletters

It is very easy to produce simple practice newsletters on an intermittent or regular basis with word processors or in-house desk-top publishing computer software mounted on standard machines. Printers or copy shops can then quite cheaply run off adequate numbers which can be distributed in the waiting room, with outgoing mail and with repeat prescriptions.

Contents of newsletters

- Notice and explanation of changes in practice arrangements
- Personnel changes
- Responses to patient suggestions
- Reminders of specific services
- Seasonal health advice
- Regular health promotion messages

The content is probably most attractive if it is in an easily read, tabloid style with multiple small paragraphs. All members of the team should contribute by writing and patients can also be encouraged to contribute. A patient participation group can become involved and volunteers from the practice list can act as editors or designers. Patients very much appreciate this sort of contact and the information provided. They gain a feeling of involvement and pride which contributes to the doctor – patient relationship.

Information leaflets

There is a large volume and range of patient advisory information available to practices freely or at minimal cost. They are useful as adjuncts to consultations but can also educate patients on appropriate self help or first line management. As many are provided by pharmaceutical houses or special interest groups, they do need to be read carefully and the appropriateness of the contents assessed before use. Local public health and health promotion organisations can also provide useful literature.

Potentially their greatest disadvantage is the profusion of number and type and resulting problems of availability and accessibility. Therefore it is best to have a small number readily and obviously available which have been approved by the practice. Patients can then be additionally directed to a point where they will always be available.

If space permits it is easy to develop a library of a wide range of leaflets, booklets, books, and audio and video tapes. Such a library can then retain information of the type which is needed infrequently or is in greater detail. There are, in almost every practice, a number of patients who would happily organise and run these sort of arrangements on a voluntary basis if given the chance.

An even greater impact on patients can be made by an in-house series of advisory leaflets. As with newsletters, they can be developed and printed cheaply and often pharmaceutical companies can be induced to subsidise their production.

Practice Annual Reports

Practices have to produce an Annual Report under the terms of service in a specified form. Both before and since the introduction of this obligation, some have often found this a useful process which helps them to maintain standards and assists in developing team cohesion. With the development of fundholding there is an increasing patient interest in purchasing plans and reports.

There is publicity and communication value in making these available to patients. It is probably sufficient to have a small number available for perusal on request in a bound form and making their availability known in a newsletter or by notice.

Practice Charters

The development and publication of a Practice Charter is a vexed issue undertaken by many as a chore of doubtful value. The overall concept of presenting a standard of service to which the organisation aspires is useful. It is preferable to emphasise the information delivery elements and express them realistically. Attempts to set unrealistic numerical targets thus raising unrealistic patient expectations will have no credibility with staff or patients and will encourage conflict and complaint.

Once prepared, highlights from a charter can be publicised by notices and in newsletters. The whole document can be made available on a request basis.

Video notice boards

The patient in the waiting room represents a captive audience. It is possible to set up and organise a video information board in a suitable place, using readily available technology which can be quickly amended or altered. Commercial organisations can undertake this, incorporating advertising and health promotion messages which can then be played on a continuous basis.

The house style

In all of these communication systems it is worth considering the development of an individual practice pattern of presentation. This can be a common pattern of presentation, layout, and colour. It can incorporate a simple logo or other practice identification, which can also be incorporated in the routine paperwork of the practice.

Such a shared style projects a feeling of competence and organisation. It also helps to engender in all the practice staff a pride in themselves and the service they deliver. The process of developing a house style can be undertaken professionally by specialised designers and modern printers can also offer advice.

Patient participation groups

One of the more problematic ways of communicating with patients is through patient participation groups. The difficulties are in finding and motivating a group of patients who are genuinely representative individually and collectively, avoiding narrow self interest. Experience indicates that they can start with great enthusiasm but it is difficult to maintain interest. Such organisations are rarely comfortable environments for patients with limited education and poor communication skills.

A newer variation is in the form of focus groups. Under the guidance of an organiser, different sections of the practice population with similar needs can meet separately.

Whichever form is used, these groups can take considerable effort to establish and maintain. Care needs to be taken that the organisation does not become dominated by the practice doctors and staff. Equally it will be necessary to ensure that the group feels its contribution is valued and acted upon. When initiating any new group it is very useful to seek the help of the local Community Health Council, who have resources for this purpose and their own networks of contacts.

Making telephone contact

The accessibility of the doctor and other team members to patients by telephone is enormously important. The vast majority of patients have the use of a telephone and expect to obtain instant access with it. Simultaneously, the doctor finds that constantly ringing telephones grossly distort consultations.

Telephone access rules

- Sufficient phone lines
- Efficient switchboard operation
- Fixed time of availability
- Accurate message recording
- Invariable returning of calls when promised

The first two elements need little elaboration, except to say that the use of unlisted lines for outgoing calls and separate Fax and Modem lines is an additional help. Service suppliers can provide a variety of sequential number and call queuing systems. Aims to answer all calls within a few rings will not be helpful if followed by prolonged periods on hold. The sensitive training of switchboard operators goes much further than the operation of buttons, and covers telephone manners and an understanding of how the practice operates and the physical place and availability of each member at a particular time.

Patients very much value knowing a specific time period when the doctor is available for telephone consultation. Properly planned – such as a period early in the morning before commencing consultation or at other times during the day – this arrangement will reduce the incidence of interruption of consultations. It can produce telephone congestion, however, unless there are sufficient telephone lines.

As an alternative, or as an addition, an efficient message taking system with return calls made to a fixed pattern, such as the same day or after a certain time, can be developed. This could be done by using answering machines but is more efficient if messages are handled by a member of staff who can also gain some idea of the reason for the call. This allows diversion to other team members if appropriate and organising the availability of records and reports prior to a team member speaking to the patient.

The use of answering machines is quite vexed and can cause a great deal of patient anxiety. When used to deliver simple messages as to call diversion they can confuse patients, and it is preferable to use automatic systems. Experience indicates that any message taking system, whether by machine or an answering service, outside the practice is likely to have a significantly higher risk of failure and needs rigid frequent monitoring and checking.

Fax systems are a useful addition to the communication tools of a practice. Two-way communication is cumbersome but direct requests such as for repeat prescriptions or documentation can be received. On occasions the ability to confirm verbal information from the practice by hard copy in emergencies can be useful. This is particularly obvious when making urgent arrangements for patient referrals.

Telephone consultation

There has always been some anxiety as to the safety of telephone consultation. It has a great deal of value as a follow-up procedure, whether doctor- or patient-initiated. Many simple administrative and organisational tasks can be conveniently handled in this way.

The additional use of bleepers and mobile phones improves the speed and comprehensiveness of availability, and responsiveness. Using these tools has greatly improved the ease of providing access out of hours. Whilst this can be regarded as more intrusive to the doctor's personal time, simple rapid reassurance and advice as to the safety of a delayed response is helpful.

All members of the team can find their work expedited and eased by telephone consultation. Particularly in the delivery of domiciliary services, the ready use of mobiles facilitates consultation and communication between team members, reducing time wastage and travel costs, and increases individual's personal safety.

Telephone use policies

Whilst the telephone as described above is an enormously useful tool, its indiscriminate use both internally and externally can cause chaos in the clinical context. Interruption of the consultation process is a major hazard, resulting in poor quality patient care. Staff therefore need clear and explicit instruction as to the circumstances when practitioners can be interrupted and by whom.

The use of message systems on computers can more silently draw information to the attention of a user as an alternative to the insistent ring of a telephone, but even this can still produce distraction and loss of concentration.

Internal practice communications

Practice has increasingly become a team effort, where there is ever-increasing need to ensure easy, safe communication between members. Message books seem cumbersome, but they do ensure that messages are not lost and they can easily include a place for the recipient to initial their collection and time. Message forms, including tick lists, especially if assisted by colour coding, have useful parts to play. In staff areas notice boards of the white board type can be useful. They can be changed daily or weekly, displaying staff availability or meetings. Many practices find it useful to use such boards for the passage of clinical information, such as recent patient deaths, dangerously ill patients or imminent obstetric deliveries.

None of these systems will work without a degree of agreement and conformity within a practice. Practitioners frequently value their idiosyncrasies and commonly refuse to conform. They can be coerced into adhering to systems by their value in avoiding income loss and by minimising patient complaints, both of which most find tiresome and upsetting. Equally there is great value in setting an example to other members of the team which will minimise the need for continuous training and reminders.

The development of written policies on communication to be used in a practice provides a useful tool for inducting new staff members. Simultaneously, the ordering of principles and practices on paper will readily bring to light methods which are impractical. If they cannot be expressed in writing easily they are very unlikely to be foolproof.

Listening and hearing

This chapter has to be concluded by a reminder that communication is always a two-way process. This means that there has to be a willingness to receive messages and information and a desire to respond suitably.

Recommended reading

Anon. *An accountability framework for GP fundholding*. EL (95) 54. Leeds: NHS Executive, 1995

Applebee K, Morgan S, Sawyer B (eds). *Croner's general practice manager*. London: Croner Publications, 1990.

Fry J, Scott K, Jeffree P. *Practice management compendium. Part 2: Organising the practice*. Norwelk: Kluwer Academic Publishers, 1990.

Heritage Z. *Community participation in primary care*. Occasional Paper 64. London: RCGP, 1994.

Hogg C. *In partnership with patients*. London: National Consumers Council, 1995.

10: Records and computers

Well-managed clinical records are a vital ingredient of good patient care and are too easily taken for granted. Therefore the organisers of vocational training have laid down minimal standards of record organisation for training practices which were originally aimed at producing an adequate briefing document for the trainee.

The same requirement of an organised and accessible record conveying all the essential clinical history serves established practitioners just as well. In this form it can be consulted more readily by other team members and will also smooth many practice administration procedures which are vital for maximising income.

The current problem

Despite the fact that general practice in the United Kingdom has flourished and grown immensely since 1911, it has done so using a system of records basically unchanged since that date. This is the minuscule basic envelope commonly known as the "Lloyd George record", so named after the politician first responsible for initiating the panel system of practice organisation.

The advantages have been its almost universal use and its small size, which reduces the cost of filing and storage. It is additionally easily transported. Whether desirable or not, it has forced practitioners to develop ingenious devices to enable it to be used.

It can be said that its poor quality is a sad reflection on the management of the service and those who represent the profession. There seems to have been a process of collusion which hopes that the problem will disappear when some new technology can take over. A small number of practices have converted to a more useful and manageable A4 record, but this has never been properly supported or encouraged.

The employers' expectation

The requirement of the regulations is that practitioners should make appropriate notes on the supplied papers and pass these via the health authority to any other practitioner taking over the care of the patient. By custom and practice it has come to be that there is an expectation that the record will also contain any other clinical information about the patient accumulated over time, so making a total birth to death medical record. Additionally it has been generally accepted that the clinical notes can be in the form of an *aide-mémoire* rather than a voluminous detailed record of every word and findings, both positive and negative.

This immediately conflicts with the fact that the service has spent many years encouraging and financing the development of computing in primary care. The investments and plans for the NHS Network for computing and communication fundamentally depend on the clinical records being available in an electronic medium based on the practice registered lists and health authorities' registers of patients.

The patient's expectation

Patients expect that their personal records should be kept on a confidential basis by the doctor and other health professionals dealing with them. The record should be openly accessible to them personally and kept in a readable form. There is an expectation that these are readily transferred, with the general practitioner having a continuous accurate, comprehensive record.

The legal advice

The climate of complaint and litigation is pushing the medical defence societies and their lawyers to recommend more extensive recording. The *aide-mémoire* is less acceptable and the recording of all actions and findings is increasingly expected. It is also expected that all documentation should be kept in the lifetime of a patient and possibly for several years thereafter.

This is therefore a pressure towards a much bulkier and less accessible record. There are additionally continued legal arguments as to the accuracy and admissibility of any electronic records.

Resolving the conflicts

These problems of a basically inadequate record system, confusion over the permissibility of electronic records, and the legal demand for comprehensives are only the start of the problem. The sting in the tail is the unresolved question of record ownership, when the paper is owned by the employer, the computer by the practitioner, and the ownership of the actual information is possibly still retained by the writer.

It remains in the patient's clinical interest, that a reasonably comprehensive record of all active and past medical details is available to facilitate current management. The key is to find a method of ensuring the maintenance of that record in an understandable and accessible form.

The whole of this process of record keeping has substantial financial implications. As records grow the proportion of space devoted to their storage increases. Physically the process of filing consumes more staff time. Simple calculations can show that in any practice several hundred records may need to be accessed in a day for a variety of clinical and administrative reasons.

Basic requirements of useful records

- Physically manageable
- Readable
- Logical
- Relevant
- Understandable
- Adaptable
- Durable

Records that are too bulky to handle or are damaged in inadequate filing areas are unlikely to be clinically useful or even consulted. Many hospitals have operated repositories of records, where old records of current patients are stored in their original form or photocopied. Physical deterioration is common and access is more difficult.

If a record is to be of use in practice it has to be one document, in a state to be handled and readily accessible at most times of the day. Readability is a related requirement, where the perennial problem of doctors' handwriting is complicated by the fading of ink, including the typewritten text, and the particular fading properties of some papers.

Maintaining records

The potential for an amorphous mass of paper where relevant information is almost irretrievably lost must be dealt with by some system of record maintenance which assists access. Obviously one of the principal methods is by ordering the information in date order. Separate arrangements including colour coding can assist in identifying sections. The currently generally available inserts for summaries and immunisation are usefully complemented by others especially developed or acquired for a practice's internal needs.

A simple method of organisation is to make all entries in date order and tag together all the continuation cards with the oldest at the rear followed by a treatment card, an immunisation record card, and a summary card. A second tag holding together similarly ordered letters and reports then completes the package. A fixed system of logical organisation similar to this would benefit single or multiple users providing that all users conform.

Pruning

The process of pruning in horticultural practice is one which facilitates new growth. Thought as to the relevance of a particular recorded or collected item leads to the difficult area of culling records. It is surprising how frequently folders contain totally irrelevant material which can be discarded without any anxiety. Much out of date administrative paper seems to accumulate.

Readability

The ease with which a record is understood depends on how easily it can be read. The physical factors such as paper and writing can often be made even more complex by the use of abbreviations and initials. When initials then become mixed with jargon which is difficult to understand, the original point is lost to all except the originator. If a dictionary has to be consulted to decode the abbreviations then they have no intrinsic value and should not be used.

Physical constraints

Any record management system needs to have a degree of flexibility which allows it to be adapted to meet changing needs. The physical storage of records needs to cope with continuous expansion and calculations as to the extra shelf length needed each year can be easily made. Manufacturers and suppliers of such equipment can provide guidance also. Simple shelving is durable providing that it is not overburdened by weight. Cabinets with sliding shelves and systems where cabinets slide or rotate bodily need efficient maintenance but have the advantage of increased compactness.

Electrically operated systems are even more dependent on expert installation, careful use and good maintenance. Again professional suppliers and fitters are invaluable advisers and can assess problems such as the weight-bearing capacity of the floor, an increasingly problematic area with converted premises, and the proliferation of paper.

Checking and culling records

Every practice is continuously registering new patients and receiving old records. A system is needed to convert the record to the pattern used in the practice. Staff are easily instructed to do the physical organisation of date order and then proceed to culling and preparing summaries after suitable training provided that they conform to clear guidelines. When computer systems are being used, the appropriate transfer and entering can be undertaken in a similar manner. It is open to the practitioner to do some or all of this process.

The same clerical and administrative process should be regularly used to keep existing records in a useful form. This may be done as a routine, working through the records alphabetically or by selectively identifying bulky or damaged records and concentrating on them.

What can be culled and discarded?

- Empty papers
- Duplicated papers
- Time-expired administrative notes
- Clinical notes made irrelevant by the passage of time

The practical current relevance of routine notes from long ago hospital follow-up is doubtful. Isolated haematological tests or urine bacteriology from years ago mean little. A letter reporting the out-patient listing of a patient for say, hernia repair, a flimsy discharge note, a formal discharge summary and a 6 week surgical out-patient report, whilst all relevant at the time, can be condensed to the single discharge summary after a year or two.

It is worth considering whether any record is worth keeping if it is also stored in another place. This is particularly relevant for items such as immunisation data, screening results, and health promotion data which is likely to be stored electronically. Many practices now have the facility to directly download pathological data into patients' comuter records. The value of additional paper storage is minimal.

All discarded material needs to be destroyed remembering confidentiality by shredding or using a specific service for the destruction of confidential waste.

The contents of useful summaries

- Consultant referrals
- Hospital admissions
- Operations
- First diagnosis of chronic conditions
- Accidents
- Births
- Major life events such as bereavement and marriage breakdown
- Significant family medical history

The summary is intended to produce a document which can be rapidly read and informs the reader that greater detail should be sought if relevant. Summaries totally recording every medical event become unreadable poor duplicates of the main record. The majority of the items can be listed in a single word or phrase.

As electronic records become more extensively used there is a parallel problem of reading to find the significant events. Simplistic data such as pathological or immunisation records can be manipulated to accessible separate screens. The consultation and diagnostic information needs to be annotated at the entry time as to its significance. The first diagnosis of epilepsy will usually be much more important than an attendance for a sore throat. The initial design of the software must recognise this problem and provide appropriate mechanisms. The accuracy and self discipline of users is also of relevance and needs monitoring.

The computerised record

A large proportion of practices have some form of computer system on which information is recorded with very variable levels of usage. This can extend from basic registration data through to the total clinical record. By the use of proper back up arrangements the computer can produce an almost indestructible total record which will always be readable.

Problems of computerised records

- Legal status and ownership
- Software inadequacies
- Lack of interchangeability
- Privacy and confidentiality
- Pace of development and obsolescence
- Costs and training

Legal work up to and including legislation is in progress on the ownership of electronic records. The inadequacies of computer software are being addressed by the universal adoption of the Read Code classification of information. Unfortunately it is not easy to incorporate within this the more vague data of the impression or suspicion type except by free text typing. Time will partly solve this problem by younger practitioners developing keyboard skills from an early age. Work is progressing on systems which can convert the spoken word into written text, but it is difficult to determine when this will be available and what the financial implications will be.

The problem of interchangeability and data transfer can be helped by the use of electronic letter boxes with appropriate conversion software. A consensus agreement or the imposition of a set format for software language and architecture will be needed to finally solve these problems. The differences of view and the continually changing abilities of both human designers, users, and technical development probably mean that some arbitrary imposition will be necessary.

The pace of change of the technology has to be addressed alongside the life expectancy of the equipment. Most equipment will start to need some replacement because of wear after about four years and a similar period will result in technical obsolescence. There is therefore a major continuing financial implication for practices and it may not be necessary continually to race after the latest equipment developments.

Advantages of a computerised clinical records system

- Produces reliable, easily used age and sex registers and disease indexes
- Readily records multiple simple items of information
- Holds clinical summaries in an easily accessible form
- Facilitates easy clinical prescribing and monitoring
- Can readily link to clinical guidelines and protocols
- Provides a tool for clinical audit
- Eases administrative processes

All the features listed in the Box are clinically useful and give added value to the process of patient care. The developing processes of electronic mail can save staff time by automatically adding data to the individual patient's record. Laboratory results are an obvious example as are results of health promotion data. An electronic record can be accessed from several points much more speedily than the paper equivalent and can have several users therefore avoiding the need for separate nursing and administrative records.

The "Links" program is an electronic mail system being promoted in general practice to simplify the patient registration processes with the health authority. The immediate advantages to the practice are limited to the rationalisation and correction of registers. More usefully, it is a building brick for simplified income claim processes.

Criteria for practice computer purchase

- Meet current health service specification requirements
- Latest technology
- Use understood language and software
- Capable of use for communications
- Capable of easy extension
- Have software support and upgrading facilities
- Available local training

These criteria are largely covered by the major suppliers with significant numbers of users. Some smaller suppliers can offer technologically interesting and sometimes cheaper solutions but this has to be balanced against whether they are sufficiently financed enough to stay in the market. The purchase is made more difficult by many suppliers insisting that software, hardware, and support are purchased as a package. This can mean paying inflated prices for some equipment when other suppliers can offer the same items at a lower cost.

As always, the buyer needs to give some careful thought to the correct compromise. Practices with greater in-house expertise may find it easier to take risks but novices are advised to use established major suppliers who do not insist on being the sole supplier of hardware.

Combining paper and electronic clinical records

Only a few clinicians are currently comfortable with abandoning traditional written notes, and they do have a significant degree of in-built confidentiality protection. This is because they cannot be easily found and read. Computers with external connections are more easily accessed remotely in a fraudulent manner, thus resulting in a loss of confidentiality and the potential for corruption and a need for enhanced security protection.

The enormous task of converting old paper records to computer probably means that, at best, only a summary and some selected items of information will be transferred by conventional clerical processes. Old records can be electronically scanned in a process similar to photocopying, producing a picture in digitised form suitable for electronic storage. Individual pieces need to be indexed to allow subsequent access. Software systems are becoming available which can additionally read and convert the scanned document thereby more fully incorporating it into the record.

New records in electronic form can be commenced, and kept well, from any current time. There needs to be an absolute commitment by the users to ensure that all the appropriate information is recorded using as much free text as is necessary.

It is possible to combine the use of both methods providing that all users clearly understand what is available in each place and the limitations of each particular class of information.

Any practice using computer records needs to have in operation methods of fully backing-up the information on a daily basis and storing that off site in a secure place. The software must also incorporate audit trail systems which allow all entries and changes to be tracked indicating the name of the operator.

Computers and the future

The world of computing and information technology is changing rapidly day by day. Whilst general practice computing is probably more advanced than in many other fields of medicine, many currently available tools are not yet in common use.

The machinery has become faster and more reliable by a combination of software advances and advanced electronic design. The consequences for the user are more easily operated machinery which is more easily adaptable to individual requirements and purposes. At a basic level colour screens combined with software tricks such as window presentations are useful. The computing power necessary for voice recognition and handwriting conversion is not too expensive to consider. That same power allows the additional presentation of moving video images with full sound facilities.

Advancing computer applications

- Communication tool
- Information source
- Education tool
- Computer-aided decision making
- Remote consultation

The first three of these are somewhat intermixed. Computers of appropriate capabilities are now easily connected with each other via telephone or radio links allowing the two-way passage of information either in text or pictorial form. At a basic level this means that, say, radiology reports or discharge letters can be transmitted from the originating source to the recipient and automatically filed against the individual patient's record. The technology to accompany this with digital passage of pictures is available.

It is an increasing problem, because of the pace of increasing knowledge, to find written texts which are up to date. Heavily used reference texts can be published in a compact disc (CD ROM) form which is easily searched and can also be amended easily on a frequent basis. They can be accessed from the desk-top personal computer or terminal and multiple simultaneous access allowed.

A step from this is using a computer to search other linked computers for stored useful information. This is the basis of the Internet and the World Wide Web but additional dedicated medical networks are also available. These networks also provide a facility to advertise effectively for information or advice.

Dedicated educational software programs are being developed. The easiest of these are attractively presented aids to patient education which can be used during the consultation or separately accessed in the patient's own home. More complex interactive educational programs are available; the use of additional sound and video capabilities enhances their effectiveness.

Computer-aided decisions

Clinical guidelines and treatment protocols are increasingly advocated to improve the effectiveness, and sometimes the economics, of medical care. These can be incorporated into systems which effectively demand conformity by refusing access to the next stage without first recording the appropriate investigation. This can then point to alternative diagnoses or treatment patterns.

Even the earliest of computer systems used for prescribing allowed the presentation of simple warnings. These have now progressed to interactions, personalised allergy warnings and clinical warnings, such as not to be used in pregnancy. The next stage systems will effectively prohibit prescribing without prior conformance to protocols and offer alternatives.

Remote consultations

The enhanced communication capabilities will allow easy transmission of moving images and pictures. The verbal discussion accompanying this will allow second opinions to be rapidly obtained in some circumstances. The projected widespread domestic acquisition of these tools may give rise to a more sophisticated type of telephone consultation in general practice. Whilst this may appear to be unrealistic, such methods would be a marked advance in the provision of care in remote areas.

Even more difficult to appreciate is the possibility of remote medical intervention. The combination of the visual and manual tools currently used in key-hole surgery and the possibility of remotely controlling them is already under experimentation in military surgery. These techniques may be particularly attractive in areas remote from extensive medical facilities or skills.

Recommended reading

Anderson RJ. *Security in clinical information systems*. London: BMA, 1996.

Anon. *Computerisation in GP practices 1993 Survey*. London: NHS ME, 1993.

Anon. *General medical services committee, guidance on medical records*. London: BMA, 1994.

Lee N and Millman A. *ABC of medical computing*. London: BMJ Publishing Group, 1996.

Pickersgill D (ed.). *The law and general practice*. Oxford: Radcliffe Medical Press, 1992.

Pringle M, Dixon P, Carr-Hill R, Ashworth A. *Influences on computer use in general practice*. Occasional Paper 68. London: RCGP, 1995.

Preece J. *The use of computers in general practice*, 2nd edn. London: Churchill Livingstone, 1988.

11: Networking for the practice benefit

Throughout professional practice there are myriad formal communications which are difficult to read and digest. Formal inspections and meetings occur seemingly without benefit to the participants. All practices need to develop methods of coping with the systems in which they work.

"Networking" is one of those terms which has come into the language and dignifies a process which otherwise could be easily disparaged or criticised. It is a useful process of gaining contact with and understanding the roles of others who potentially have an influence over significant aspects of practice activity. The obvious first stage is the need to understand the roles and power of other people in their own organisation.

Potential benefits

- Information and education
- Finance and resources
- Guidance and help
- Influence on decision making

Lack of information can be likened to a form of blindness and its acquisition is part of the totality of education. Whilst it can be comforting, in the short term, to function as though the rest of the world does not exist, the lack of current information can be very damaging to practice functioning. An acceptance of the need to keep in touch will usually avoid the risk of significant resources being lost, or never acquired, due to ignorance. Similarly, knowledge of new or different patient services can advance the patient's interests and minimise unnecessary work.

The process of obtaining help or guidance to solve difficult issues will not be useful unless it is preceded by a knowing who to turn to. Rarely does any organisation have within itself all the skills needed, and good networks give cheap and easy access as well as a degree of advance warning.

Clinical networks

- The Primary Health Care Team
- Local practitioner colleagues
- Local community health services
- Specialist colleagues and secondary service providers
- Social services – social workers and care workers
- Housing officers and wardens
- Local occupational health services

All those listed in the Box have a relationship to the smooth functioning of clinical work in any practice. The roles and the work of the members of the Primary Health Care Team have already been discussed in a previous chapter, but it is worth emphasising the need for the doctors to work at the maintenance of the links. This involves time for face to face contact and a listening process that goes beyond the exchange of clinical information and includes gaining an understanding of their anxieties and needs.

Because local practitioner colleagues and the community services can be seen as competitive, there can be a tendency to believe that contact should be minimal. In reality there are many clinical and organisational reasons for valuing good relationships. Examples of this are where local practices need to cooperate for off-duty cover or where spouses of patients need to be simultaneously investigated for infertility. Understanding the strengths and weaknesses of local community services can facilitate decisions as to which services practices need to provide for their patients.

All of the others listed have the capability to make the individual practitioner's life both easy and difficult. A developed understanding of their responsibilities, capabilities, and the personalities involved is generally more likely to result in harmony and cooperation. This extends from the local home help providing useful information to the ready telephone access to hospital colleagues for advice or help. The noting and use of names with an understanding of the individual's status in their own hierarchy does help, despite the fact that the staff of some organisations change frequently.

The health authority

Over the past few years there have been enormous changes in the authorities with which practitioners interact. This has culminated in 1996 in unitary commissioning authorities which now both manage the contract with practitioners for primary care and are also responsible for arranging secondary care. Whilst they do not directly control the purchasing activities of fundholders, they have a significant role in monitoring and budget setting.

There is no one standard pattern of organisation within these bodies and there are additional differences between the provinces of the United Kingdom. It is therefore essential to know the important local names and titles and gain some understanding of their activities.

Health authority major players

- The authority chairman
- Non-executive authority directors
- Health authority executive directors
- Chief executive
- Primary care director
- Medical adviser
- Pharmaceutical adviser

Generally speaking, the chairman is a political appointee for a period of four years and is remunerated on a part-time basis. He or she bears the ultimate responsibility for the functioning of the authority and its delivery of the objectives set by government either directly or via the NHS Executive. Each is aided by a group of non-executive directors who are also part-time and remunerated, appointed for four year periods, and usually from a less overtly political background. There has been a deliberate policy of appointing persons who have some experience of management in other fields. A number of general practitioners and other contractors such as dentists and pharmacists have been so appointed but there is no statutory right to representation. Most authorities have at least one non-executive member from a nursing background who is not an employee.

Usually about three or four senior officers are also appointed as executive directors on a full-time basis. These will always be the chief executive, the finance director and a medical director, who will often come from the public health discipline. In many authorities the executive responsible for general practice is not necessarily at this senior level and therefore may have difficulty in advocating its needs and problems. Even further away from the top table can be the specialised medical adviser for general practice and the pharmaceutical advisers. Despite this, it is helpful to try to get to know these people and understand their individual range of authority.

Local management

A variety of subordinate organisations may exist below the authority level. They will frequently have a geographical basis or alternatively a specialised role. This can be a very crucial level with regard to secondary care contracting issues.

Within the organisation will be a number of other individuals who can be just as useful and informative and who are likely to be more easily accessible. Making friends with the senior assistant can ensure rapid access and can often save time if only at the level of redirecting enquiries or explaining procedures.

The provider organisations

Practices and practitioners need to relate to multiple providers. There will usually be one or two local principal trusts but practitioners often refer patients to a large number of providers, some of whom partially or wholly offer services on a private basis. They need to know the employers of the other primary health care team members who are not on their own payroll.

Fundholders need to make formal contracts with providers. Prior to reaching that stage, or even the earlier process of negotiation, there is a process of information exchange. This has enhanced value conducted on an informal basis and the whole networking process can be used to obtain comparative information.

Provider organisation major players

- Chairman
- Non-executive directors
- Executive directors
- Business managers
- Medical director
- Human resource managers
- Clinical or service managers

The trust chairman and non-executive directors are similarly appointed to those of the health authorities. Rarely are clinicians of any sort appointed to non-executive positions, although universities, and therefore medical faculties, are represented when the trust has a major teaching role. The executive directors always include the appropriate chief executive and head of finance. Another director will usually cover the needs of the physical infrastructure and the service functions such as catering.

There is usually a clinical director, who is a consultant employed by the authority, functioning part time in this role. Most, but not all, clinical directors will be appointed for their ability to deliver an acceptable level of leadership of their colleagues and act as their representative.

All providers are major employers of staff, the majority of whom will be nurses. This seems to be the justification why the most senior employed nurse manager often has the title of human resource director. This may include the whole of the trust's personnel management function. The senior nurse manager should logically be a trust executive director.

The business manager is usually a trust executive director who has the responsibility to organise its contracting process. They have a mixed role of liaison with purchasers, negotiating contracts, and organising the administration processes of charging and income collection. This person will usually wish to develop close relationships with fundholders making major contracts for services. The very largest providers may choose to undertake this process via a number of business managers, functioning on a locality basis or by clinical specialty.

There is considerable variation of organisation within provider organisations at the level below the board of directors. General practitioners will need to use local knowledge or networks to understand the pattern. Sometimes the head of a particular service may be a clinician or alternatively a nurse. Occasionally a non-medical person can be the named manager with a varying degree of rationality. For community services the lesser roles may be based on geography or professional discipline. All of these service heads will usually work closely with the business managers and relate jointly to practitioners. This is particularly relevant to fundholding and commissioning activity.

Private service providers

There is no simple way of understanding the structure of these organisations. The terms consultant, manager, director and chief executive can be used indiscriminately. Sometimes this can be confusing when looking at the detail of clinical services. Close study of their published literature and direct questioning will be needed.

Other primary care providers

It is easy to forget about the other contractor services which are important to patient service. Practices need to understand the range and nature of services provided by local pharmacists, dentists, and opticians. Physiotherapists, chiropodists, and podiatrists are active in all localities. Personal links and contacts will add value to clinical care. There is additional scope to carefully exchange clinical information on individual patients.

The whole range of providers of alternative medicine present a slightly different problem. It is certainly important to understand what they are doing or even claiming to do for individuals. It is not so easy to develop relationships which include the passage of individual patient information.

Community Health Councils

Unfortunately these bodies have become labelled with the concept that they exist solely to organise complaints against practitioners. In reality they are desperate to relate to primary care and understand how practices function. Careful communication and meeting with their officers will usually be rewarded with a much higher degree of understanding and support. They are usually as knowledgeable about local problem patients as are practitioners. As allies they can assist in the process of manipulating change in provider services.

The primary care led NHS

The changed health service has brought with it an opportunity for practitioners to have a major influence on its style and organisation. To exercise this power it is necessary to understand the developing structures within which practitioners operate and to learn how to communicate with them and within them.

Exercising joint influence

- Fundholding groups
- Total fundholding projects
- Locality purchasing schemes
- Locality commissioning schemes

The differences between these schemes are mainly about the extent to which they actually hold, spend, and account for the necessary finance or alternatively simply advise. All of the schemes involve representatives of practices, usually doctors but frequently additionally practice managers, regularly meeting together to develop common views on local services. Whilst much is done in formal meetings, the addition of informal networking will facilitate joint understanding and policy development. The subsequent negotiation processes with health care providers will be enhanced by prior networking.

Community orientated primary care

This is another new concept which is developing in general practice. Involved in it is the idea of being more responsive to the demands of the community and an increasingly positive approach to seek the appropriate accurate opinions of the patients on the form and structure of services. A better developed understanding of sociological factors in the pathological processes can be combined with closer working relationships with the community social work teams and voluntary bodies. Apart from the more obvious patient participation work, this involves practitioners supporting and informing voluntary organisations, especially those of a self help type. It can amount to a system of encouraging and facilitating patient self advocacy rather than the more traditional medical model. The general practitioner needs continuously to be maintaining contacts to understand the values and aspirations of other organisations in the field, whatever their origins.

Networking, persuasion, and manipulation

These processes are inevitably mixed together and do not need separation. They are integral to negotiation and should be used with deference to the local political climate.

Rules for networking

- Use formal and informal opportunities to meet
- Honest discussion
- Be able to listen and respect others' views and perspectives
- Maintain telephone accessibility and return calls
- Record and remember with discretion
- Remember to reciprocate

A courteous approach combined with a considerate style which accepts the scope and limitations of others' knowledge and authority is essential. The addition of a forced pattern of socialisation or excessive adulation will not improve an already poor relationship. Genuine friendships are inevitably used and will often arise from networking but they are not compulsory. For the reduction of stress and facilitation of relaxation an entirely different networking system is needed, which is outside the scope of this text.

Recommended reading

Gregson A, Cartlidge A, Bond J. *Interprofessional collaboration in primary health care organisations*. Occasional Paper 52. London: RCGP, 1991.

Ham C. *The new national health service*. Oxford: Radcliffe Medical Press, 1991.
Henry S, Pickersgill D (eds). *Making sense of fundholding*. Oxford: Radcliffe Medical Press, 1995.
Irvine D, Irvine S. *The practice of quality*. Oxford: Radcliffe Medical Press, 1996.
Wilkin D, Hallam L, Leavey R, Metcalfe D. *Anatomy of urban general practice*. London: Tavistock Publications, 1987.

12: Choosing a practice

The ability of any individual to choose his or her practice will be determined by a number of different factors but probably the most important is the number of current vacancies. If the applicant is limiting his or her choice to a particular area or type of practice, then the ability to choose added to competition from other applicants can lead to disappointment. It is unwise always to expect that a perfect position will necessarily be available. A sensible applicant should be also looking at prospective practices in terms of how they are likely to be changeable or alter in the future and what effect they themselves, as individuals, can have on that process. If there is a current labour shortage resulting in few applicants, the aspirant is increasingly better placed to determine his or her own terms.

Why choose me?

Any person about to apply for a job has to assess what he or she has to offer which makes success more likely. This is a two-way process also dependent on the job on offer.

Self assessment

- Training
- Experience
- Qualifications
- Special medical interests
- Sex
- Language and communication skills
- Personal factors

Obviously all applicants will be trained, but there is no doubt that some training practices provide appreciably different experience. The applicant trained in an inner city is less likely to hold the necessary knowledge suitable for remote rural practice and vice versa. Simultaneously, the extent to which individuals have been exposed to the administrative aspects is variable.

The possession of multiple qualifications may not be essential but the MRCGP is increasingly regarded as desirable or even a prerequisite. The accumulation of additional diplomas in paediatrics and obstetrics is less important, but they do carry a certain prestige and can impress prospective employers and patients. Almost invariably prospective employers will wish to appoint applicants already qualified for child surveillance and minor surgery. The possession of a certificate in family planning is almost essential and experience sufficient for admission to the obstetric lists is frequently requested.

Additional interests and knowledge which brings the opportunity of extra remunerative activity will usually be welcomed. Clearly any employment offer may be targeted with an applicant of a particular sex in mind but not overtly expressed. A locality may have a predominant or significant ethnic mix where language skills are useful additions. The area of communication skills includes an appreciation of whether the applicant shares and understands the local culture and dialect.

An extrovert who likes a fast life style is probably unlikely to be happy or meet with approval in rural areas. The relative anonymity of a large city will meet some individual's personal requirements better.

What do I want?

The simplistic answer of a fast car, not much work, and a large income is not likely to create the best impression, even if it does have a ring of truth and is probably in the subconscious of all.

The ideal job

- Partnership or not?
- How large a practice?
- Geographical location?
- Fulfilling personal ambitions?

The traditional view has always been that a partnership or the sole practitioner status is the norm. This is being challenged as a partnership can hinder personal mobility and flexibility and will involve significant heavy and prolonged financial commitment. The attractiveness of a salaried post as an assistant or associate is therefore increasing. Similar criteria for selection should apply, with the need for a partnership agreement replaced by a contract of employment.

It is probably unwise for the newly trained practitioner to aim immediately for single handed practice. Whether by application to fill a vacancy or the starting of a new practice, working alone demands significant experience and preparation and is discussed below. A large group practice may have some advantages in a wider range of facilities and skilled staff, but this can be outweighed by increased communication and organisational problems.

There can be a greater level of competition for posts in some of the more attractive areas. A desire to practice in a limited area can result in a lack of vacancies and a temptation to accept an unsatisfactory post.

The career patterns and objectives of spouses and domestic partners are of great significance and must be taken into consideration. The ability to pursue or develop special clinical interests, whether new or old, is important. Equally the need to access varieties of recreational facilities cannot be lightly ignored.

Finding vacancies

The steps outlined above will set the scene for the next stage of deciding which vacancies are worth pursuing. It is not always easy to find out what is available, as a variety of means of recruitment are used by practices.

Searching for vacancies

- Advertisements
- Personal networks
- Trainers' contacts
- Health authority primary care managers
- Self advertisement

The way in which advertisements are placed can be just as significant as the detail contained. The sole use of free space in some medical newspapers or on notice boards presents an entirely different image from the elaborate layout in expensive journals directing enquiries to a recruitment agency. It is difficult to understand the thinking of those who use the anonymity of box numbers, but the motives of those who choose to advertise in non-medical journals with limited sectarian readership is more obvious.

Some practices entirely restrict their search for applicants to names passed to them informally on their own networks. The aspirant must therefore seek to keep in touch with a wide range of personal contacts who may have valuable information. These contacts should usually include trainers and previous employers both in the hospital service and in practice.

Local primary care managers frequently know when practices are intending to seek new partners, as may prominent local practitioners. This can be particularly useful when an applicant wishes to stay in a particular geographic area. Self advertisement in journals or on notice boards may be helpful but is done more effectively by working in an area as a locum for a period of time.

Making the application

It is always wise to follow the requests of the advertisement speedily. The temptation to bypass the specified route may create the wrong impression, although a personal approach complementing the formal application can be helpful. Unfortunately many do not specify closing dates for applications so it is wise to assume that the window for application may be quite short.

Key stages

- Initial contacts
- Letter of application
- Curriculum vitae
- Presenting references
- Relevant investigation
- Expressing enthusiasm
- Varieties of interviews

An offer of further information should always be pursued or, in the absence of an offer, direct enquiry made of the practice to elicit adequate information. A good impression is then made by a letter of application which relates the applicant's qualities and aspirations to the known or supposed needs of the practice.

The curriculum vitae which accompanies this should be informative but not so elaborate as to deter a busy reader. A useful guide might be a limit of two pages, thus ensuring that the whole is read by the recipient. The detailed content of a résumé must always be accurate and specific. It should include some information as to the applicant's experience and involvement outside of professional practice. A brief indication of career and personal ambitions is a useful element.

Referees should only be stated with their prior approval and chosen carefully to avoid embarrassment. Some prospective employers will insist on a reference from the last or current employer, which can cause difficulty. An honest explanation of the particular problem in providing such a name until after a job offer is made, or of the nature of a dispute, may help, along with the offer of an alternative.

The interview

A wise applicant will prepare for the interview process by careful discrete investigation of the practice and its neighbourhood. Time spent in gaining an impression of how the practice functions, the locality, and other local health services will facilitate any type of interview. Such knowledge will convey a degree of enthusiasm to prospective employers as well being useful in itself.

The actual format of the interview or multiple thereof can vary enormously. Because most practices appoint additional doctors infrequently, and are then potentially committing themselves to complex agreements, the process can be quite prolonged and appear inept or clumsy. If the applicant has not met all the prospective colleagues by the final interview stage, this will indicate the possibility of problems.

Because the prospective practice can be apprehensive about the whole process a number of variations are beginning to appear. Recruitment consultants can be used to assist in the preparation of shortlists and assessing the personalities of the applicants.

Candidates may be asked to make presentations on a set aspect of practice activity or their personal qualities.

There continues to be the vexed question of the social type of interview accompanied by an invitation to the applicant's spouse to attend. These "trials by sherry" are likely to be resented, especially if involving the spouses of existing partners. Direct refusal to cooperate is unlikely to be helpful if there is a wide field of applicants. Alternatively it can be said that the practice which cannot make a decision on its business and professional life without such an event is probably dysfunctional. Such a formalised process is quite different from the normal social courtesies of offering help or refreshment.

Meeting prejudice

It is unfortunately true that employment legislation, with its protection from sexual and other forms of prejudice, does not apply to the making of partnerships. Covert expressions of racial or religious prejudice can sometimes be anticipated by the placing of advertisements and the unreasonable emphasis in interviews on matters of ethics.

Obviously all forms of prejudice are regrettable and to be avoided. The intensity of a partnership relationship probably always means that there will be a greater emphasis on personal factors than in the case of employees. Despite overt signs of prejudice the applicant will have to decide personally whether to pursue the vacancy. There is a fine line between the assertion of rights, however laudable, and entering into a partnership which by its nature is dysfunctional. Where other applicants are known, they can be informed, allowing them to make appropriate decisions.

Dealing with an offer

Before responding to an offer and during the selection process, it is essential to ensure that all the crucial information has been obtained and understood. The appropriate documents should have been seen and inspected at leisure, with professional advisers if necessary.

Checklist of minimum information

- The reason for the vacancy
- The practice's expectations of the new partner or employee
- The workload commitment and duty rosters
- Anticipated future changes
- Holiday, sickness, and maternity leave arrangements
- Financial arrangements, both current and anticipated
- Current practice agreement

The deliberate withholding of any of this information should be treated with caution, as should loose verbal agreement to clarify detail after acceptance. Doubts at this stage are best discussed with a third party, such as a former trainer or a trusted friend in general practice. Compromise between the ideal and what is available will always be necessary, but too much compromise is a recipe for long-term unhappiness. Negotiation on the offered terms has not been common but a good applicant in an area with a labour shortage does have scope to negotiate improvement.

Coping with failure

Coping with disappointment and rejection

- Reviewing personal deficiencies
- Changing approach
- Maintaining enthusiasm

It is always possible to blame all failure on the intended employer or the other candidates. Failed candidates can quite reasonably ask informally why they have not been accepted and can find the explanations helpful. The possibility of excess ambition or inadequate preparation should always be part of a review. Further training or experience could well improve the chances at the next opportunity.

Whilst it is natural always to seek to join the perfect established practice in a perfect place, there is only a limited availability. It can therefore be useful to review personal expectations and consider the extent to which an applicant may be able to influence change in the future in a practice advertising a vacancy. The imminent retirement of a partner or the acquisition of new premises could well provide an opening for large and exciting change.

Even the most successful do not succeed at every challenge and rejection is not the end of the world. There is an overall inadequacy in the number of available trained practitioners and patients will supply an endless amount of work!

Succession to a single-handed practitioner

Taking this route brings a number of additional problems which potentially produce a heavy workload. The appointment process may be accompanied by a need to simultaneously acquire premises and staff. The patient load might well be problematic, with an unstable or falling list and a legacy from different preceding clinical policies. Additionally local colleagues can be antagonistic or even obstructive in their attitudes, particularly affecting arrangements for out of hours care.

In making such an appointment the health authority will probably wish to see firm evidence of planning to cope with these issues. The extent to which the practitioner wishes to work with that authority and the support it offers is crucial.

It can appear easy to switch from the problems of partnerships to the freedom of independence. The price is almost certainly a heavier workload, especially initially, and a greater level of responsibility. A total range of individual skills and knowledge will be needed in the organisational and managerial field and clinical support may be minimal.

Starting a new practice

The majority of new practices, whether single-handed or not, start because of partnership disputes. The effects of this on patient loyalty are quite unpredictable, with consequent insecurity for the doctors. It is not wise to assume health authority support as they may view the situation as an extra drain on their resources and detrimental to primary care team establishment and function. The problems are similar to those of an individual succeeding to a single-handed vacancy with the addition of an extra degree of local professional animosity.

There are occasional situations where local practices are prepared to encourage and support the development of a new practice. This will usually be where existing practices consider themselves overloaded and are not prepared to expand. This can be linked with housing developments or the geographical and demographic constraints of a locality. In these circumstances support by suggestion to patients and by the action of the health authority can be available. In some circumstances specific additional inducement allowances may be paid.

The practitioner starting a new practice totally alone finds that the most important problem is the length of time needed to attract sufficient patients for financial viability. Simultaneously, the availability of health authority allowances is dependent on a minimum list size. This means that to undertake this process significant additional financial planning is needed. It may take several years and alternative additional work may need to be done simultaneously. The availability of such additional work may depend on the physical relationships to local hospitals and care has to be taken to ensure 24 hour availability whatever the list size.

Changing practices

There has always been a cynical and disparaging view taken of practitioners moving between practices. This is unfair, as much movement is dynamised by the individual's social and personal needs. It can be a logical career development move and all practices can probably benefit from the regular infusion of new blood, both experienced and newly trained.

It is grossly unfair to assume that an individual moving between partnerships is inevitably a difficult person. The decision to move is not taken lightly and it may well be to the advantage of both patients and partners that individuals do not feel themselves constrained to persist where they are unhappy.

Recommended reading

Meads G (ed.). *Future options for general practice.* Oxford: Radcliffe Medical Press, 1995.

Williams S. *Making best practice better.* Frome: Publishing Initiatives Books, 1994.

Willis J. *The paradox of progress.* Oxford: Radcliffe Medical Press, 1995.

Index

9 780727 910370